So God created man in His own image, in the image and likeness of God He created him; male and female He created them. And God blessed them and said to them, Be fruitful, multiply, and fill the earth, and subdue it [using all its vast resources in the service of God and man]; and have dominion over the fish of the sea, the birds of the air, and over every living creature that moves upon the earth. And God said, See, I have given you every plant yielding seed that is on the face of all the land and every tree with seed in its fruit; you shall have them for food. And to all the animals on the earth and to every bird of the air and to everything that creeps on the ground—to everything in which there is the breath of life—I have given every green plant for food. And it was so. And God saw everything that He had made, and behold, it was very good (suitable, pleasant) and He approved it completely. And there was evening and there was morning, a sixth day.

Genesis 1:27-31 (Amplified Bible)

whollyfit

wholly fit
body & soul

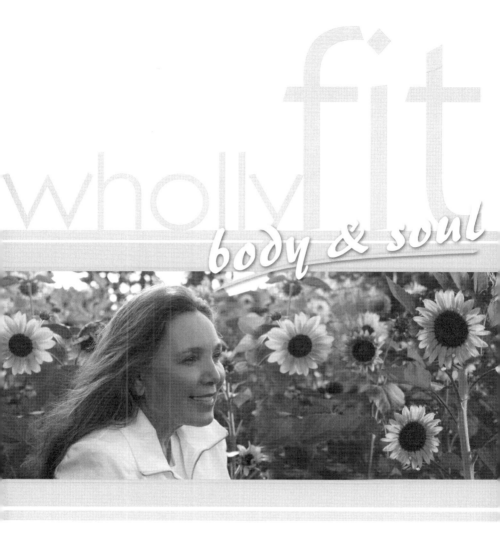

NANCY GRANDQUIST

Wholly Fit Body and Soul copyright 2009 by Nancy Grandquist.

ISBN 978-0-9747414-8-2

Book cover design by Angela Carrington of Inspire Media, LLC.
www.inspiremediallc.com

Photography by Charity King of La Bella Vie Photographie
www.labellaviephotographie.com

Interior design by Cara Davis Creative Services
www.caradaviscreative.com

Disclaimer: This book is not intended to take the place of medical advice from a trained medical professional. Readers are advised to consult a physician or another qualified health professional regarding treatment of their medical problems. Neither the publisher nor the author takes any responsibility, should there be any negative consequence to any person who reads the information in this book and then chooses to apply medicine or herbs to themselves or to others.

❀ About the Author ❀

First and foremost, let me say that Nancy Grandquist has to be one of the most interesting and fabulous mothers any girl could have. Whether she is writing the latest doxology song at 2 a.m., or working on her latest manuscript, there is always a new project in the works. I have often teased my mother that at the age of 105, she will be in her wheelchair asking me for my opinion on her latest endeavor. My poor father had no idea what he was getting himself into. Thankfully, he is her biggest fan, besides me. There is no limit to her abilities. Although she speaks into the lives of thousands of women around the world, she knows the value of the simple moments in life, and cherishes pouring into the lives of those closest to her. You can find my mother knee-deep in chicken manure searching for eggs, just because my daughter, Emma, loves the adventure. Life was meant to be lived, and Nancy Grandquist lives it to the fullest, and you can't help but experience it with her. As you read the pages of this book, you will discover for yourself her obvious passion about living life as a whole person – body and soul. You too will be Wholly Fit if you take this book to heart and ask God to give you the strength and fortitude to make these very necessary, life-changing steps.

Heidi Grandquist-King

Nancy and her husband of 40 years, Richard M., live in the San Francisco Bay area where they pastor The Rock Church. She has four grown children, six grandchildren, two sons-in-law, a coop full of chickens, a Cavalier King Charles Spaniel named Bingley, and a Persian cat named Henry. She travels internationally, speaking and inspiring thousands of people with her transparent heart. She is also a prolific songwriter and author.

❀ Dedication ❀

This book is dedicated to my dear brother, David. Even in the very last days of your beautiful life, you inspired me with your courageous heart. Now, every time I see a startling, red sunset, a freshly plowed field, a fence loaded and leaning over with fat, juicy blackberries, or when I hear the strum of a guitar, the hum of a harmonica, I think of you. I see your face and hear your voice and I miss you. We all do. You planted the seed in my heart to write this book.

To Taylor, Josiah, Joshua, Emma Love, Sophia and Isabella and those grandchildren yet to come: I thank God for the blessing of you. My deepest desire is for you to find the pure path to living a balanced life. I love you to the moon and back. Nan.

Acknowledgements

Thank you, first, to my God and creator. You are the reason I live. Next, I want to express my deepest gratitude to those people in my life who continually encourage me to follow my heart.

Thank you, Richard M. Not only are you my husband, but you are my very best friend. We have shared much love, laughter and happiness over the past 40 years. You remind me every morning that life is a gift and that I must live it wisely. I love you with my whole heart.

Thank you to my beautiful family for your patience and understanding while I spent many, many hours on this book. To my church family and friends all around the world, you are precious to me.

Thank you, Michelle Hibbert, Barbara Nickens, Marcia Lang, Tracy Jorgensen and many others who helped me in my research. Your input was invaluable to this project.

Thank you, Charity, for traipsing through the dirt fields of the late October sunflower crops. You make a photo-shoot so much fun!

Thank you, Krystal Mayville, for your brilliant mind and prodigious gift of finding the best way to succinctly communicate one of the passions of my heart. You are wonderful. You understand exactly what I want to say and you help me to express it clearly with strong conviction. You are incredible and I never want to write another book without your help and humor.

To Heidi King, you always seem to put the icing on the cake with your quick mind and your ability to capture the very essence of my words.

Thank you, Cara Davis, for your eleventh hour formatting and template design. You are a life saver!!

Thank you, Mother, for being my teacher and mentor and for inspiring me to learn how to cook wonderful foods. I love you. You are the best mother any girl could have!

TABLE OF CONTENTS

INTRODUCTION

It breaks my heart to see people make bad food choices. They are making themselves sick! That is why I have decided to start the Wholly Fit Revolution. I am totally committed to helping you find that ultimate level of health and balance in your body and soul. All I need from you is a made up mind that you are going to DO this, despite the obstacles in your busy life. I want to empower you to search out the foods that will heal your body and seek out the truths and concepts that will revitalize your soul.

There are four basic principles you need to grasp as you begin your journey toward finding a vibrant, happy and healthy life. (1) Think of food as energy, both positive and negative. (2) Be the real you. (3) Open your life to positive change; and (4) Stick with the plan.

Who else should be expected to be the vanguards of holistic health and natural healing? The children of God, of course (those who are created in His image)! We who teach the necessary disciplines and restraints for guarding our temples and our souls should be the ones! We, as an American society, have looked to the healthcare system as the answer and provider for our every medical need, but we should also be well studied and informed in the avenues of holistic and naturopathic wellness. I am acutely aware of my miniscule, limited qualifications for communicating the vast amount of health information that is available today. However, as I have gleaned from many resources, I have become passionate about finding the healthiest ways in which to live a Wholly Fit life. We are advocates of finding wholeness and restoration for our spiritual souls. Should we not also seek to be as whole physically and emotionally? I believe our

Lord wants us to be just as fervent in the preservation of our whole being. On that basis, I have included with this book an exercise CD for your benefit. It has five music tracks, is approximately 40 minutes long, and provides the perfect music for a fun and exciting workout. I promise that once you hear this music, you will not be able to stand still, so get up and GET moving!

Nancy Grandquist

1

the Scoop

O kay, raise your right hand and solemnly promise to tell yourself the truth, the whole truth, and nothing but the truth. Remember, GOD is going to hear you!! Say this out loud: "I am beautifully created. I am wonderful and I can't help it because God made me perfectly."

If I could, I would disarm every magazine rack that caters to writers who do nothing but critique, criticize, and compare people from the crook in their nose, to the space between their front teeth, to the split on their big toenail. I will scream if I have to look at one more title on THEIR magazine that tells me to practice a particular exercise which will make my waist magically shrink down to a size 2 by simply holding a position for 5 minutes!!

I do not want to leave you men out, soooo if you guys are sick and tired of being bombarded with pictures of Godzilla-like males with blood veined, Ripley's Believe It Or Not steroid-induced muscles, then come join the rebellion. I am OVER it! Now, if YOU are ready too, we have a lot to share. I can already feel a sense of camaraderie and we have barely started. So go get a decaf cuppa, (that's what my Australian friends call a cup of coffee) scoot your chair up, put your

1

feet on pause and stay awhile. We have got some work to accomplish, some laughs to share, and some memories to make. Are you ready?

The Bible says a double-minded man is unstable in all his ways. This speaks to me about the importance of having clarity in our thought processes. We must discipline the thoughts that would love to run rampant in our brains. I want you to think right now about the areas of your life that steal your energy, bog you down and leave you feeling wrung out, tired and defeated. Hopefully you are not thinking about your spouse, because if you are, then we have already hit a brick wall. This book is not about fixing relationships. It is about restoring our physical bodies and walking down the path to better health. I will say, however, that when we feel better, we are able to think more clearly and perhaps with that new clarity we will become a bit wiser in our relationships. Imagine yourself waking up every morning, vibrant and ready to face life and its challenges. Not to mention, you will actually be able to step into those clothes you wore twenty years ago without feeling and looking like you are wearing the little spandex exercise rig that belongs on your wiener dog.

Now, I want you to take a deep breath and then slowly exhale. Good. Now do this two more times. Feel the oxygen moving through your lungs, then pulsing to the tips of your fingers, continuing throughout your entire nervous system, cleaning your arteries, strengthening your muscles, and purifying your blood. All of this happens in just a few concentrated, deep breathing movements. When you inhale you should imagine your lungs hugging your heart. When you exhale, you should be able to feel the fullness of your lungs as they touch your kidneys. In this one deliberately simple act, you have already begun to work out the negative stress factors that steal your vitality! More to come on this subject later! Baby, get ready to get your life back!! I am going to expose a dark and dirty little secret that we ALL know about ourselves, yet none of us are willing to talk about it. Here it is: we constantly excuse ourselves from being fit because we believe that we do not deserve to spend the much needed time it takes to care for ourselves. You think there's an elephant in the room now? Well, you had better wake up right now, Honey, because an entire herd of elephants just came in and they are not going away!

One huge roadblock on the way to our fit selves is that we tend to follow the crowd and order the biggest hamburger with four patties, extra cheese, and an extra large side of fries. While some of you may say that this is one of our favorite American pastimes, I prefer to instead call it one of our sacred cows. I seriously believe that we need to throw that golden calf into the fire and have a bona fide meltdown! I am not trying to be Debbie Downer, but I have studied enough to know that those super sized French fries happen to be arterial atomic bombs! In addition, if you had any idea how some of the slaughter houses process red meats, you would take a solemn vow to never drive your family through a fast food hamburger joint again. There are currently meat packing plants that are vigilant about the way the meat is prepared but they are few and far between.

Another practice we need to perfect is learning to read and understand food labels. We must be careful in this learning process, however, because we can easily spend an entire afternoon in one aisle of the grocery store while our families sit at home staring sadly at their empty dinner plates and wondering whether they will see us (or their dinner) before nightfall. It would amaze most people to discover how much a true portion size is. For instance, when the package says 8 chips or 1 cup of popcorn, it means exactly that. It does NOT mean the entire bag. Pay attention now. I want to help you with your portion sizes.

- 3 ounces of meat equals the palm of your hand (minus the fingers!);
- 1 to 2 ounces of nuts equals one cupped hand;
- 1 ounce of meat or cheese equals the size of your thumb; and
- 1 cup or 1 medium whole fruit equals your fist.

As a general rule, a serving size of milk is only one cup. Whole milk should be given only to growing children and, unless you, as an adult, desire to grow some more, then I do not recommend you drink whole milk. Additionally, 2% milk is recommended for teens, as they are still growing, but need less fat than whole milk. For adults, it is suggested that we drink 1% or skim milk. It is also imperative that we consider and then actually practice consuming foods that are highly nutritious and that do not have excessive amount of fats and sugars.

—∿—

You might as well take a number and sign up for a heart defibrillator right now.

Would you give your beloved child a glass of poison? Of course not! Why, then, would you give them diet drinks filled with mutant-making, tumor-multiplying, fraudulent-feeding ingredients? Whew! That could give your brain a charley horse. I suggest that we start a revolution - a new trend. Break the mold and lead the pack! Just say no to the grease, no to the sweets, and especially NO to the midnight meals that we do not need. Yes, I said that!! We do not need them!! Instead, drink some water with freshly squeezed lime or lemon or drink your favorite herbal tea. How about eating a leafy green salad with olive oil and vinegar for dinner? Now there is a novel idea (especially if you are one of those people hooked on dousing your salad with two cups of ranch or blue cheese dressing). Honey, you might as well take a number and sign up for a heart defibrillator right now. If you insist on consuming calorie-loaded salad dressings dripping with so much fat that they could be used for a blood thickener, then I strongly suggest that you dip the end of your fork into the side of the dressing rather than drenching your lettuce leaves with it. This is a prime example of how we can balance our thought processes by making good choices. Think whimsical thoughts - light and airy - not forklift thoughts!

America is one of the most generous countries in the world when it comes to portion sizes. If you do not believe me, take a look at that 20 ounce slab of meat hanging off the side of your plate, along with the baked potato heavy-laden with sour cream, butter, and chunks of bacon. I have often observed patrons at American-Chinese restaurants gobbling down fattening orange peel chicken, sweet and sour pork, fried rice and chow mein. Meanwhile, the cooks and employees are sitting back in the kitchen eating healthy Bok Choy, steamed brown rice and slices of watermelon. Go figure.

Okay, now that you can see where I am going with this, I want you to understand how extremely vital it is for you to make up your mind. You must choose to be healthy and never look back. Once your mind is made up, everybody else needs to LOOK OUT! Wild horses will not get in your way. The scripture declares that as a man thinketh in his heart, so is he. We have to start thinking and saying to ourselves, "I am worth the time, money, effort and everything else it takes to be healthy and feel good." You need to identify whatever it is that makes you want to eat the wrong things all the time. Many of us eat for comfort. I happen to call it emotional eating. Whether you choose to call it drama eating, theatrical eating, party animal eating, or another comfort idea, it needs to be controlled and come under submission! Our son, Richard is studying in the medical field and has become very aware of nutritional value. One of his favorite healthy snacks is frozen green grapes and it has become mine too. Instead of reaching for potato chips, I now go to the freezer and get a couple of grapes. Now that may not impress you, but please understand that I am a "chips and dip" kind of girl and I have made a landmark turnaround in my diet! And yes, just to set the record straight, I occasionally hide in the pantry and smuggle Cheetos into the pocket of my housecoat. Nobody is perfect, you know.

It is important that we find the appropriate keys to help us strengthen our resolve and establish the fortitude we need in order to make the right choices whenever we start having those out-of-control food cravings. We must make a declaration that we are giving God full control over every aspect of our lives, including an authentic visualization of every morsel of food that we put into our mouths. There are a lot of things we eat that cannot be labeled as a nutritional food and we will talk about this later.

Our heavenly father cares about the smallest details in our lives, including the number of hairs on our heads and in our noses. I know that was gross, but it is important for you to understand that IF God cares about the very intricate details of our lives then we must honor him by caring enough to look after ourselves. PLEASE PAY ATTENTION to this next sentence. YOUR VALUE AND YOUR WORTH ARE FAR BEYOND YOUR COMPREHENSION. You may have some serious doubts about this concept and may even believe otherwise. However, you cannot argue with God because He will win the argument every time. I want to share some profound truths from God's Word. They are heavy duty, mega doses of affirmation. I want you to get a wide-eyed view of all that you are (the way God sees you) and all that you are about to become.

You are the apple of His eye.
You are His beloved.
You are His precious jewel.
You are anointed.
You are His bride.
You are blessed.

You are His companion.
You were made fearfully.
You were made wonderfully.
You were made for a purpose.
You were made to reign with Christ.
You are blessed.

You will judge angels.
You are filled with His glory.
You are wrapped in His righteousness.
You are the salt of the earth.
You are the light of the earth.
You are blessed.

You are set apart.
You are protected.
You are a warrior.
You are an overcomer.
You are healed by His stripes.
You are blessed.

You are washed in his blood.
You are forgiven.
You are entitled to His throne room.
You are His child.
You are precious.
Oh, yes, and you are so blessed!!!!

Hopefully you have been given a glimpse of the beauty that surrounds your life and the rare and exquisite frame of all that makes up who you are. You do not have to do one thing to make yourself valuable. Just your mere existence in this world makes you a treasure. You are one of a kind. Love yourself, respect yourself, and believe in yourself.

I feel so sad for those of you who are chained and fettered to the obsession of never being thin enough (perhaps even battling with anorexia or bulimia). I am worried about what you are doing to yourself. Richard M. and I think Mr. Bingley, our Cavalier King Charles Spaniel, needs therapy/doggy counseling. He has displayed several symptoms that lead us to believe he has a serious eating disorder. Early one morning around 6:00 a.m., I awoke to hear Richard M. talking to someone. I got up to see who in the world would be at our home at that early hour and as I walked into the room with my counseling hat firmly in place, prepared to listen to someone pouring their heart out, I was instead surprised to see our little Bingley sitting on Richard M's lap. His big, brown eyes were looking straight at his master. The two were fully engaged and having a heart-to-heart "Let's be real. No more pretenses" talk. This is where the doggy counseling fad started.

Normally, we are quite diligent about watching the amount of food that Bingley eats because these types of dogs are known to die from heart attacks due to their obese nature. I recently walked into the library/pool table room to see Bingley backing out of a discarded pizza box that somebody had put in the fireplace (pizza boxes make great fire starters). When Bingley saw me walk in, he acted very pensive and sheepish. As I bent down to look closely at him, I spotted half of a piece of cold, leftover pepperoni pizza dangling out of the side of his mouth. Richard M. and I talked to Bingley again, but I have a feeling it went in one ear and out the other. Bingley also has a problem with loyalty. He runs off every chance he gets. Mostly he runs down the street to the grocery store, but most recently he ran away to the neighbor's house to join their huge Super Bowl party. A few days before this, we had taken Bingley to the dog groomer who put a football scarf around his neck. My guess is that Bingley got into the Super Bowl spirit, although it was probably more about the food then the game for him. Here is my point to all of this. Do not act like our little Bing. Tell yourself the truth. Be loyal to yourself and to the ones who love you so much. You may think it sounds weird for a dog to be a closet eater, but I happen to think it is weird for humans to be closet eaters. There is nothing worse than hiding, being disloyal and lying about your health and happiness.

There are a lot of frustrated, depressed people who desperately want to feel better and who beat themselves up because of the evil BATHROOM SCALE. I know people who carry their scale around, guarding it as if it is a sacred artifact from King Tut's tomb. They weigh themselves on it every few hours to make sure they haven't gained an ounce. What I really want to say to those obsessive compulsive people is this: "Chill out! You are doing yourself a huge disservice by weighing yourself all day long." As a matter of fact, weighing once a week is the suggested and healthy way to keep track of your weight.

There is nothing worse than hiding, being disloyal and lying about your health and happiness.

Look, I do not care if you want to lose 10 pounds or 100 pounds. I truly believe you can do it with Gods help, but I do not think we should even talk about dieting until we get our minds set on positive, encouraging, joyful thoughts! First things first. The most important thing is to get your body healthy, humming, and happily functioning the way God intended it to be! Here is some food for thought (fat free food). The Bible says our bodies are temples and are designed to be filled with God's spirit. It is against God's law to defile our bodies. Our bodies do not belong to us, but to God. If we know these things are from the Word of God and they are true, why do we not live and believe them? We often hear about the terrible effects of using marijuana and tobacco as well as the inevitable and devastating price that is paid for abusing alcohol and other drugs, but what about the catastrophic consequences of stuffing ourselves with food that has zero nutrition? What about the huge volumes of food we ingest until our buttons blow apart? It is astounding the amount of food that we consume. I am afraid we are guilty of gluttony. Gluttony, My Dear One, is a sin. Ouch, that hurt my feelings! Webster's definition of a glutton is a riotous eater and one that eats and drinks in excess.

NOW, HOLD UP JUST A SECOND! For all of you little skinny things out there who eat the entire kitchen and never gain an ounce, I have one question for you. Why are you reading this? Skip the book and go straight to the Wholly Fit Exercise CD. You would not understand a word I am saying. Besides, you make me (and everyone else) want to scream when you tell us about your chronic obsession to try and put on some weight, but that it is just not possible. Please, please, please have a little compassion and shut your mouth.

It is human nature for us to be oversensitive and easily offended, so I hope that as you read this book, you will understand that my heart is prayerfully considering the things that I am writing about. I was speaking at a ladies' conference one evening and felt compelled to share my thoughts on the way we have neglected to care for our bodies. I tried to be so careful and I talked about myself first and how I love to cook and bake and that I love to eat even more! I poured out my heart to those incredible women even though I was a bit apprehensive. I shuddered to think I might offend or hurt someone. The next morning as I was addressing the conference, I looked out and saw a young woman in the audience who reached into her purse, pulled out donuts and began to eat them, one right after another! When I looked at her, she caught my eye and stuck her tongue out at me. I had to contain myself because I wanted to bend over and howl with laughter. I spoke with her close friend after the session and explained that I wanted to talk to her friend and make sure she was not upset. I was assured, though, that everything was fine. She further informed me that her donut-eating friend was a staunch advocate of greasy, fried foods and that I would never persuade her otherwise. Oh well! So much for my indelible influence! My hope is that I will manage to provide a better influence within the pages of this book than I did at that conference.

I must tell you that I come from a long line of southern cooks, (Mean Mama kind of cookin'). I'm talking about fried chicken with a bowl of butter and chives to dip it in, mashed potatoes, cream gravy, fried corn bread, biscuits and sausage gravy with fried potatoes, fried eggs, and double-dipped, crushed cornflakes-fried French toast. We also believed in seasoning our collard greens and I am not just talking about salt and pepper. We would put in a huge slab of salt pork and the entire kitchen sink if it called for it. Plus, every time August rolled around, the Gravenstein apples were picked, peeled, and pared so that we could build a pie from scratch. But that is not the end of our pie tale. My "skinnier-than-a-bone-rack" mama also taught me to make a vanilla sauce (which will be on Heaven's dessert bar) that goes on top of that angel flaky pie crust which is then finished off with a big scoop of homemade vanilla ice cream. Hopefully you get my point. I have gone through rehabilitation for my food addictions. Food rehab for me is an extremely disciplined fast from all food which is totally different than a fast unto God and I will cover this subject later. I have shared with you this brutal personal confession so that you will understand how vulnerable I am to making bad food choices.

Wow! When I typed those words I thought I heard my grandmother yelling at me. She has been gone a few years now, but along with her memory I can almost smell the pinto beans and white bread with fresh butter from Daisy, my granddad's cow. Yep, my brother David and I loved to get out the bucket and get yummy, fresh, organic milk right from the source. You may be smiling and making fun of me now, but please understand that milking a cow is an art. You really should give it a go sometime.

What I want you to see is that with all of my homegrown roots, food represents just about every aspect of my life. I have had to readjust the way I think about breakfast, lunch, dinner and the in-between snacks. I am sure you have heard the old adage, "Eat breakfast like a king (queen), lunch like a prince (princess) and dinner like a pauper." In other words, do not eat large amounts of food prior to retiring for the evening. This is going to look insurmountable to some of you, but please do not let it be. I try to eat basic and simple whole foods because I believe that is the way we were meant to eat. I also love to eat fruit in the morning because it is an anti-inflammatory and a great start to a new day. I especially love watermelon (with seeds still intact. The vitamin potency is diminished when you eat seedless watermelon). I also enjoy blackberries, blueberries, mango, papaya, oranges, apples, grapes, and bananas. In my opinion, blueberries are the best since they are very high in antioxidants.

I try to eat basic and simple whole foods because I believe that is the way we were meant to eat.

I also have a juicer and make organic juice. I use carrots, apples, fresh ginger, beets, and whatever else I may have on hand. I try to eat living food. EAT OATMEAL TOO! Oatmeal will actually lower your cholesterol. We should probably talk about the way you eat your porridge (that is the term for oatmeal which Goldie Locks and the Three Bears and my friend, Jena, from Sydney, Australia have dubbed it). My family crowned me The Oatmeal Queen of the West because I would add butter, brown sugar and heavy whipping cream. However, this is a gigantic fat ball waiting to gather around your waist and keep you from ever bending over and touching your knees or being able to tie your shoelaces. Here is a better way. Try using low fat milk and maple syrup or else use some raisins, dried cranberries or sliced strawberries in it. It tastes so good and is SO much better for you!

I like to keep a handy supply of organic almonds, cashews, and macadamia nuts. Walnuts are excellent too, but I happen to be allergic to them. When I buy dried fruit and vegetables, I choose those that are totally natural without sodium or preservatives. I am a huge advocate of purchasing whole grain breads, pastas and cereals, but the best bread you can eat is sprouted and it says so on the package! I was having a conversation with a woman from the Netherlands and she was shocked at how much white flour and sugar Americans consume. In the Netherlands, their diet consists mainly of wheat flour and dark rye breads. Even their pastas are made from pure, organic ingredients (semolina, durum flour and aquina flour). I understand that in some parts of the country it is difficult to find stores that carry natural foods, so my suggestion to you (if you fall in that category) is to be adventurous and buy organic whole wheat flour and just bake with it!

Try making stir-fry with as many leafy green vegetables as you can fit in the pan and add some water chestnuts for crunch. Instead of brown or white rice to accompany your stir-fry, try quinoa, which is a protein, instead of a carbohydrate, and just as yummy! It is very easy to overcook your vegetables, so please stand there while they cook. I start with chopped onions and then add garlic into the olive oil. Did you know that olive oil actually cleans your arteries? Wow! Together we are learning some very valuable and important food ideas. I want to make this plain and simple so that you get it. Are you getting it yet? Eat organic. Eat your vegetables and especially eat as many raw fruits and veggies as you can. Fruits and vegetables should be 80% to 90% of our daily food intake. Fish, chicken, meats and pastas should be 10% to 20%. A simple way to help you plan out a balanced meal is to visualize your plate covered with mostly vegetables and a palm-sized serving of protein. This is critical to the building and maintenance of a strong immune system which will help your body fight off sickness and life-threatening diseases.

I went out to my garden recently, picked 2 cucumbers, washed them and ate them right there on the spot. Now, I do not expect you to run out and plant a garden (although it's really not a bad idea when you consider how expensive groceries are) but please think green. Think anti-oxidants. Think quality of life. Think Popeye the Sailor Man…Yes, think spinach!!

You should eat salmon, cod, or whitefish at least 3 times a week. There are other recommended types of fish, but I do not like sardines, herrings, and all of those other stinky varieties. I am sure they must be incredibly good for you because they smell horrible! If you want to try them out, be my honored guest. Just don't cook them in my kitchen. It is also a great idea to eat 10 servings of tomatoes per week (provided your stomach can handle the acid). Cook them. Boil them. Eat them raw. Barbecue or grill them or throw them in your spaghetti sauce. Something about a cooked tomato puts it into the next category of wonder food. Here is a heads up for you men. Recent studies show that eating tomatoes in any form, even on your pizza, helps to maintain a healthy prostate. One last thing. Don't forget the yams and sweet potatoes. They are soooooooo yummy and healthy for you.

2

lifestyle in Motion

The way in which we live our daily lives has a tremendous affect on our health. If we ignore basic health laws, we cannot expect to live life to its fullest. It really is up to us to study and search out the best ways to live our lives so that we are able to maintain a healthy and productive lifestyle. On my parent's homestead is a beautiful pasture which has known many seasons. Some seasons yield crops and brilliant sunflowers. Other seasons yield an amazing wonderload of pumpkins that have grown big enough to accommodate Cinderella's carriage. Yes, we even have enough mice for many footmen. In the middle of that same pasture sits a 1947 musty-smelling, green Plymouth truck. We are very much infatuated with this ancient piece of automobile history. For years, everyone in the family has talked about how incredible it would be if the truck were refurbished with all the bells and whistles. It would definitely be worth a small fortune, yet there it remains, doors flopping open, rusted chrome, and leather seats frayed and decayed to unidentifiable fragments. It has, over time, become a haven to stray cats and the occasional possum who loves to dine on my mother's chickens. It has also provided shelter for some rather obnoxious skunks and scary, silent spiders with webs that lay claim to any innocent creatures looking for a layover in their travels. As you take time to absorb the mental picture of the abandoned truck, please realize that I may have just described you. Everyone around you loves and adores you beyond measure and your worth is invaluable. Yet you remain a paralyzed promise of potential. I think it must make our Heavenly Father sad to see us with so much sickness and in so much pain with so little energy to do the things He has called us to do and the things that we desire to do. We must discipline ourselves by eating only enough to be strengthened and then stop! Instead of living on the edge of diabetes, high blood pressure, clogged arteries, strokes and heart attacks, we must take charge of our bellies!

There are obviously situations we cannot avoid, no matter how conscientious we are about our diet and exercise. For instance, if we are invited to dinner at someone's home and they have cooked up a big country meal with fried foods sitting on every corner of the table and seven desserts to choose from, it would be rude to turn up our nose at the meal, pull an apple out of our purse and nibble on it as everyone else partakes in the feast. As much as possible, though, we should make responsible choices. We are fearfully and wonderfully made. God impeccably designed our bodies with an incredible blueprint so that we would be restored and rejuvenated and so that our bodies could heal themselves. However, our bodies can only take so much abuse and neglect before they break down and become weakened and diseased. Imagine if you will that we have all been given a basket to carry around every day and inside that basket is a small amount of fruit, bread and pasta. As the days pass us by, we keep adding additional and unnecessary items to the basket until it is so heavy that we have difficulty carrying it anymore. However, if we begin to remove items from the basket, we will begin to feel better and the load is not as heavy. This is the analogy of how our body responds when we carry extra pounds. Likewise, as we lose the extra pounds the body becomes resilient and begins to heal itself and feel better. It is up to us to obtain all the knowledge and instruction that is available to us and use the wisdom to develop a healthy and productive lifestyle.

God gave us a wonderful brain, although sometimes I wonder how much we use it! It seems at times a strong possibility that we have put it into semi-retirement or sent it on a long vacation. We should learn, grow and develop our ability to make appropriate choices. We cannot be swayed by peer pressure. We have the power of choice and it is up to us to choose wisely. Remember, attitude equals outcome and it is all in the choosing!

3

body and Soul

The Balance and Diversity of All that We Are

Man, by God's design, is made up of body, soul and spirit. Our spiritual nature needs and desperately desires to worship something in order to fill the empty void that stretches to the very depths of our soul. In our world today are objects of worship, such as sports arenas and Hollywood. Society finds itself fixated on these personalities that are merely mortals, but what man deeply and innately desires is a relationship with his creator. That relationship was corrupted by Satan in the Garden of Eden, but God later brought redemption through Jesus Christ and the finished work of Calvary.

It is a wonder beyond measure to know Jesus Christ and to worship Him in Spirit and in truth. Oh what bliss to know Him as our father. He wants us to live in His presence and to have a relationship that brings the most beautiful fellowship. There is perfect peace and a continual flow of joy that prevails even through the most difficult times. We know our father wants to give us the very best because we are His own children. How wonderful it is when we give ourselves fully to him who started the work and will be faithful to complete it in us. He desires for us to prosper and enjoy good health. Our communion and commitment to loving God and others brings assurance that God is for us and even when He requires us to walk through difficult times, He intends nothing but the best for us. He desires for us to prosper and be continually blessed in all aspects of our lives - body and soul.

We must have a healthy perception of ourselves in order to live life to its fullest. The Bible says in Galatians 5:14, "Thou shalt love thy neighbor as thyself." How can you possibly love others if you do not have a healthy love and respect for yourself? I do not mean that you should have a mirror fetish, nor do I want to leave you with the impression that we should be totally self-absorbed. There is something really stinky about a narcissistic personality. This type of person only thinks about how wonderful and perfect they are and that the world is fortunate to have them. I have met a few people who fit this description and they are so sad. Nothing is as pitiful as a person who cannot see past the end of their own nose, thinking the entire world revolves around them.

One of the walls in our dining room is mirrored from top to bottom and it has always been quite interesting to watch people as they eat and observe themselves in the mirror. Over the years, there have been people so entirely interested in their own reflection that they literally stared at themselves in our mirror until their food grew cold. I'm not suggesting that we jump on the narcissistic bandwagon but I strongly believe it is important that we all have a good self-image. How can we influence others in a positive way if we do not value our own lives? We need to look at ourselves. Is there room for improvement? Are there things we need to change? Then by all means, we must go change! We must remember who we are in Christ Jesus and remember our invaluable worth.

People are constantly swayed by fads and trends in the magazines and movies. Sadly, there is an epidemic of very thin women who have no idea who they are inside. They, in turn, are affecting the younger generation and we now have this huge identity crisis. Because people do not know themselves, they cannot love themselves. A woman recently spent over $50,000 on cosmetic surgery because she so badly wanted to look like Angelina Jolie. What a tragedy it is that our society has become so enamored with Hollywood. What happened to relaxing, being a whole person and celebrating the uniqueness of our own lives? We are products of God's perfect design and we should feel confident in that fact.

We should always strive to better ourselves. For example, when the enemy comes in like a flood and whispers words of condemnation and pours condescending thoughts into our minds, we must resist by remembering who we are in Christ and our invaluable worth. We are higher than the angels. We are the express image of God. We are created in His likeness and yes, we are beautiful in His sight. How ridiculous it would be for a prince to disclaim his rightful place in the kingdom by denying his royal bloodline. Even more ridiculous, as God's children, we tend to forget in moments of weakness that we have been empowered by the creator Himself to become the sons of God. One day we will rule over angels. They envy us and desire to be like us. Why should we live below our privileges? When Satan and his angels sinned, God threw them out of Heaven. However, when man sinned, God came to earth, wrapped himself in flesh, and became our Savior and Redeemer. We are unmistakably more important to God than even the angels of Heaven.

4

staggering Statistics

Wе have an epidemic of overweight, obese and sickly people in our nation. This should **not** be the case in the body of Christ. We should lead by example by practicing discipline in our eating habits and exercising the self-control to stop eating when we know we are supposed to stop. Remember, I am preaching to myself, so please do not get mad at me and assume I am pointing my finger at you. We are in this together. If we have no self-control or discipline in the physical realm, we will never have it in the spiritual realm! Philippians 3:17-19 says, "Brethren, be followers together of me, and mark them which walk so as ye have us for an ensample. For many walk, of whom I have told you often, and now tell you even weeping, that they are the enemies of the cross of Christ: Whose end is destruction, **whose God is their belly**, and whose glory is in their shame, who mind earthly things." I do not want to get too heavy here (no pun intended) but we need to look at the role of nutrition and what it means to have a properly balanced diet.

According to the IHRSA/ASD Obesity/Weight Control Report, 3.8 million Americans weigh over 300 pounds. The average adult woman weighs in at 163 pounds, and 400,000 Americans (mostly men) fall into a super-massive 400+ pound category. The U.S. Surgeon General's report declared that obesity is responsible for 300,000 deaths every year. Approximately 40 years ago, research statistics showed that the percentage of obesity in America's population was at 13%. By approximately 20 years ago this had risen to 15%. Within approximately 15 years this number increased to 23% and by the year 2000 the obesity progression in America had reached an unprecedented 31%! It is now 2009. You do the math!

—ᗰ—

Did you know that you could be obese, yet thin?

Obesity is defined as having a Body Mass Index of 30 or greater. Body Mass Index is found by comparing height and weight. Obesity may put you at risk for developing heart disease, asthma, sleep apnea, high cholesterol, type 2 (insulin dependent) diabetes and hypertension, just to name a few. Here some other mind-boggling facts from the Center of Disease in the United States. 65 million people are overweight. That accounts for 8 out of 10 people over the age of 25 years old who are overweight. 40 million are obese and 3 million are morbidly obese. Did you know that you could be obese, yet thin? Obesity refers to what is happening on the **inside** of your body by taking into account the high fat content versus the small muscle content of your body. These components must be proportional to your height, frame and weight.

The World Health Organization and the U.S. National Institute of Health recommend using the Body Mass Index (BMI) to determine our ideal weight range. To calculate your BMI, you will need to fill in the blanks by answering the following questions. It may be helpful to use a calculator for addition, multiplication and division, but if you are anything like me, I still use my fingers.

To Calculate BMI

Your weight in pounds _____. (Be honest, now!)
Your height in feet and inches_____.

- **Step 1:** Convert your weight to kilograms by dividing your weight in pounds by 2.2.
- **Step 2:** Convert your height to total inches by multiplying your height in feet by 12.
- **Step 3:** Convert your height in inches to meters by dividing the result of step 2 by 40:
- **Step 4:** Square the height in meters by multiplying it by itself.
- **Step 5:** Divide the weight in kilograms by the height in meters squared (divide the result of Step 1 by the result of Step 4).

BMI Zones

- **BMI of 25 or less** = normal healthy range. HOORAH!
- **BMI of 26** = overweight and flirting with danger. I AM WORRIED ABOUT YOU!
- **BMI of 27 to 29** = dangerously overweight. I AM CALLING YOUR MOTHER!
- **BMI of 30 or greater** = obese. THAT'S IT. I AM CALLING THE FAT POLICE!

When you read this next paragraph, you will most likely break out in a nervous rash. Get this. For every additional pound you gain, your body creates one mile of additional blood vessels to nourish that pound. For example, if you are 20 pounds overweight, there are 20 miles of extra vasculature in your body. One pound equals approximately 3,500 calories. For each pound of body weight, we need approximately 15 calories per day to maintain. A 120 pound woman would need to consume 1,800 calories per day to maintain her weight. A 200 pound man would need 3,000 calories. To lose a pound, we need to eliminate 3,500 calories from our diets. If the man and woman both went on a 2000 calorie per day diet, the man would lose a pound every 3 ½ days, while the woman would actually gain weight at the rate of approximately 1 pound every 17 days until she reached about 133 pounds.

Here is some SUPER SIGNIFICANT AND SERIOUS STUFF you should know about your cholesterol:

- Less than 200 mg/dL is desirable and generally puts you at a relatively low risk of coronary heart disease. Please have your cholesterol levels checked often or as your doctor recommends.

- 200-239 mg/dL is borderline-high risk. Your doctor will evaluate your levels of LDL (bad) cholesterol, HDL (good) cholesterol and triglycerides. It is possible to have borderline-high total cholesterol, HDL (good) numbers with normal levels of LDL (bad) cholesterol balanced by high HDL (good) cholesterol. Your physician may create a prevention and treatment plan including lifestyle changes, eating a heart-healthy diet, and exercise. Depending on your LDL (bad) cholesterol levels and your other risk factors, you may also need medication.

- 240 mg/dL and over is high risk and may put you at *twice* the risk of heart disease as people whose cholesterol level is desirable (200 mg/dL). Again, your physician may create a prevention and treatment plan including lifestyle changes, eating a heart-healthy diet, and exercise. And of course, depending on your LDL (bad) cholesterol levels and other risk factors, you may also need medication.

The lower your LDL (bad) cholesterol, the lower your risk will be for a heart attack and/or stroke. In fact, your LDL is a better gauge of risk than total blood cholesterol.

Generally, LDL levels fall into these categories:
Less than 100 mg/dL = optimal
100 to 129 mg/dL = Near Optimal/Above Optimal
130 to 159 mg/dL = Borderline High
160 to 189 mg/dL = High
190 mg/dL and over = Very High

- The average range for a man's HDL (Good) Cholesterol is 40 to 50 mg/dL. The average range for a woman is 50 to 60 mg/dL. An HDL cholesterol of 60 mg/dL or higher offers some protection against heart disease. The higher the levels of HDL (good) cholesterol are the better off you are. Low HDL cholesterol (less than 40 mg/dL for men, less than 50 mg/dL for women) puts you at a higher risk for heart disease. Being overweight and having a sedentary lifestyle (watching your bananas ripen) can result in lowering HDL cholesterol. To raise your HDL levels it is recommended to maintain a healthy weight and get at least 30 to 60 minutes of physical activity at least three times a week.
- Triglycerides are a form of fat. Those with high triglycerides often have a high total cholesterol level, including high LDL (bad) cholesterol and low HDL (good) cholesterol.

The ranges for triglycerides are as follows:

Normal = less than 150 mg/dL
Borderline-High = 150-199 mg/dL
High = 200-499 mg/dL
Very High = 500 mg/dL

It is all about balance. We must balance the food we eat with daily physical activity. We must eat whole grains, vegetables and fruits. We must eat low fat and we must watch our sugar and sodium intake.

CHEMICAL CALORIES

I was recently introduced to the term, "Chemical Calories" by Dr. Paula Baillie-Hamilton, M.D., PhD., who studies human metabolism. She points out that the additives, chemicals, pesticides and other growth hormones used to genetically modify our plants and animals also make **us** grow when we consume these products. Additionally, these chemical calories are claimed to alter our hormone balance and damage our metabolism. We really should be militant about avoiding these foods. We all want to shop at Wholly Fit grocery stores, but that often seems to require funds from our entire pay check. So, if you buy regular non-organic veggies and fruits, please give them a good scrubbing in order to remove these chemicals. Grocery stores now sell a fruit and vegetable spray that washes away the chemicals. You can find it in most produce sections. I know how difficult it is to incorporate these changes into our lifestyle. In fact, it seems impossible! I was sitting in an airport recently, waiting for someone to pick me up and had just been informed that they would not be there for three hours. I had been flying all day, had not eaten one thing and was juggling three suitcases. What do you think I did? I completely unloaded the vending machines. However, after reading the labels (chemical calories) I decided to call it a fast day even though I was ravenous! Writing this book has obviously done a number on my head. I would rather starve than eat the junk that will set me up for all these scary health problems.

5

happy, Healthy

and Wholly Fit Children

I t is time for us take our children's health into our own hands. They have become physically and emotionally unhealthy. As children, they have no idea that the stuff being pushed in their faces will eventually lead them to many unnecessary problems. So, here is my recommended antidote. Shut down the video games and DVDs. Throw that idiot box out into the street. Help your kids find their imaginations again. Maybe they have never had one. We must take responsibility! We should be the inspirations for their creative bend. Although it seems easier to plant them in front of a movie with a bag of popcorn rather than thinking of something inventive and constructive for them to do, it is **imperative** that we spend quality time building and nurturing our children. We need to remove the "media parent" and step into the **real** parent role so that we can enjoy the rewards of seeing them grow and become well-balanced individuals.

It takes a huge effort on our part as parents to inspire our children to eat the right foods. The June 23, 2008 issue of *Time* magazine was dedicated to the health and welfare of our nation's children. Some of the statistics were pretty mind boggling. Kids are becoming seriously sedentary. Many of them are spending at least three hours a day in front of a TV or computer and many of our schools have lost their funding for physical education.

In the 1950s, kids drank three cups of milk for every one cup of soda (okay, I was born in the 50s and I cannot remember very many times when a soda came into our home). Today, children drink an average of three cups of soda to one cup of milk. The inevitable is happening. They are loading up on calories with virtually no nutrients and I cannot even bear to think of what is happening to their teeth while all this sugar wreaks havoc on their pearly whites.

There has been a rise in obesity among our children from 19% in 2004 to 90% in 2008. Here's the problem. We allow them to overeat and gorge on their food rather than just eating until they feel full. Our early ancestors back in the days would kill a wild boar and then eat until they could not eat anymore. Why? Because they never knew when the next meal was coming or where it was coming from. Now, fast forward to 2009 and here we are, still eating like they did (except that we do not have an excuse because the majority of us do not HAVE to chase after our dinner). As a result, we have become fat and our children are on the verge of outsizing us. These very young, obese children have developed sicknesses associated with people in their 40s and beyond. Type II diabetes is now being diagnosed in our young teenagers. Also shocking is a warning by health experts that the current generation of children may be the first in American history to have a shorter life expectancy than their parents. "The more overweight you are, the worse all of these things will be for you…" reported acting U.S. Surgeon General, Steven Galson. "When you are talking about morbidly obese kids, 0% will grow up to be normal weight adults."

—𝔪—

Parents can fight this bulging battle and lead by strong example.

As parents, we can turn the destructive tide of obesity in our kids by demanding healthy snacks and lunches in the school cafeterias. If it took thirty years for us to get in this bad shape we should be able to turn it around by reversing the epidemic back to the point where we have good, sound, healthy children. I have watched my daughters become almost militant about the food and snacks their children consume. Our youngest daughter, Kate, teaches preschool children and is constantly aware of what her toddlers eat when they are in her care. She has had many serious discussions with parents about the food choices for their little ones and has staunchly refused to allow junk food in her classroom. She has instead created an environment that encourages and affirms the children to eat "yummy, yummy in my tummy" health foods. She emphasizes the brilliant color of green in broccoli, the bright orange in carrots and she makes up fun games and stories about all of the different "wonderfoods" that God grew in His garden just for us.

Parents can fight this bulging battle and lead by strong example. Teach your children to develop healthy eating habits and encourage physical activity at an early age. Make your kitchen a sanctuary. Ban all soda (regular and diet) from the house. Declare war! Clear out your refrigerator and pantry of junk food. Make sure you have healthy snacks available. Praise your children when they choose healthy foods and when they are physically active. Make sure the family has a healthy breakfast before they leave the house. No excuses! Be active as a family.

If your kids are obese or overweight, it is critically important to listen to what they say about their weight and their self-image. Empathize with them. Tell them you love and accept them, no matter their size. Never, never, never use food as a punishment or reward. An overweight child should not feel forbidden from or deprived of food. That can trigger food hoarding (closet eating) and emotional problems. Make fast food an occasional adventure – NOT a way of life.

Put wonder veggies in spaghetti sauce, vegetable stir fry, bean burritos and soups. Make healthy fruit smoothies for your children. Involve your children in the grocery store excursion by asking them to pick out fun and interesting vegetables and fruits. If your children are old enough, invite them to help you cook. It makes them feel important and helps them appreciate the foods they are eating. They love to help clean, peel, and cut up vegetables. Plant a garden and as the vegetables grow, let your children pick and eat them. Serve freshly cut veggies and fruit as an afternoon snack.

Please, please, please eat your meals together as a family at the dinner table. Turn off all electronic media. Enjoy the food, conversation and laughter. Provide structure for a healthy family. Set rules and boundaries for your children to follow. Do not get in the bargaining game with them by saying, "If you eat your vegetables I'll give you some dessert." If you do this, you are diving headlong into a food power struggle and nobody will win in the long run. Last, make sure you involve the *entire* family in healthy eating habits. Never single out an overweight child by making him/her eat differently than their siblings. This is extremely unfair and sends a message to the overweight child that they are a bad child and are being punished.

SEIZING THE MOMENTS

My kitchen was organized, spotless, and squeaky clean one day, when to my pleasant surprise my middle daughter, Heidi and her husband, Chad came through the front door followed by their two little ones (two of my grands) who ran in screaming, "Yahoo!! Let's make some cookies, Nan!!!" Now, I know that soon and VERY soon, they will be grown up and their lives will be filled with many incredible and interesting opportunities. But for this brief moment, 2 ½ -year-old Emma and 5-year-old Joshua think that I am one of the coolest people that ever existed. So, I brought out the mixing bowls and measuring spoons and before anyone could blink an eye, egg yolk was sliding down the cabinet doors and I was crunching sugar between my toes with every step I took. WHEW!! You talk about flour power! It was like a mighty cloud descended right down upon us. Then came the expressions of pure delight from those two little faces when we took the cookies out of the oven. I instructed them to stand guard while I stood and blew on the "too hot to frost yet" cookies. When I finally

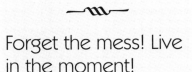

Forget the mess! Live in the moment!

said, "Okay!" they dove headlong into the frosting bowl and WOW, what a confectionery sugary shindig we had. As ceremony dictates, we then moved to the couch with our milk glasses filled to the brim (where we always have at least one spill). Our plates were piled high with warm, delicious, decadent cookies and our favorite storybook was tucked firmly under one of their chubby little arms.

When these moments come, I savor the sweetest reward of my life as I look at their cherub faces smeared with cookies and frosting and smiles that I will forever frame and hang on the inside of my heart. Forget the mess! Live in the moment! Our lives are far too uptight. We are stressed out and shackled to our schedules and deadlines, crowded freeways, telephones, text messages, and e-mails. We have got to slow down and take time to revel in the moment. We must enjoy the moment HERE and NOW!

It was another beautiful day and I was torn. My children and I were outside and in awe of God's great masterpiece. They wanted me to stay and take a walk with them, but I needed to get on the road as I was 1½ hours away from my appointment which I could not afford to cancel. However, I finally caved into their pleading, "Mom just stay a few more minutes!" We began walking and soon came to a bend in the road. Right in front of us and through the trees was the most picturesque and pristine lake in Santa Rosa, California. Immediately a million memories and pictures flashed through my mind of other lakes, beaches and oceans I had visited. I do not know what came over me, but the next instant, my shoes were flying as I ran down the hill with reckless abandon and dove headfirst into the water. I came up sputtering and dying laughing and as I walked out of the lake I noticed a lifeguard. I honestly did not see him sitting high and lifted up on his lifeguard stand. He started clapping his hands, whistling and then screaming, "Bravo!!! Well done!!!" The other innocent bystanders then joined him. Never for a second did I expect a standing ovation, nor did I even take the time to consider that there were other people on that beach.

When I walked back to collect the shoes that I had so gracefully kicked high into the air, there stood my poor, darling children in a state of shock. My daughter, Heidi, said, "Mom! Isn't that your good silk skirt?" I said, "Uh Huh." Chad said, "Mom! Don't you have to be at your appointment immediately?" I said, "Uh Huh!" Joshua said, "Nanny! You jumped in the lake and now you're all wet!" I said, "Uh huh." And then we all died laughing. By the time I got to my appointment, my clothes were fairly dried out and slightly smaller than they were prior to my jumping in the water and my hair-do was officially "washed-up" so to speak…or is it washed out? At any rate, this is a hilarious memory and of course my children love to tell the story. We learned a very valuable and important lesson that day. Take the moment by the tail and do something! Live the moment! Silk will dry out. Hair-dos can be revived, but the chance to experience life will pass us by much too quickly. So laugh! It is good medicine. Hug your spouse, your kids, your family, your friends, and your church family. Talk to people. Talk to strangers. Be warm. Be friendly. Be real. Change your world. You can make it happen. Just MAKE it happen.

6

essential Nutrients

Vitamins, Fats, Carbohydrates, Proteins, Minerals and Fiber

"The Doctor of the Future will give no medicine but will instruct his patients in the care of Human Frame, Diet, and Cause/Prevention of Disease."

Thomas Edison, 1902-03

VITAMINS

If you are unsure you are getting the vitamins you need, then I suggest that you talk to a nutritionist about putting you on a daily vitamin regiment appropriate to your body's needs. I drink a daily vitamin cocktail every morning which consists of two ounces of Monavie, one tablespoon of Total Omega 3.6.9 (which consists of organic flax seed oil, fresh catch fish oil and pure borage oil). I add one tablespoon of aloe vera juice and one tablespoon of Nature's Answer liquid hair, skin and nail vitamin into that drink. I also take a multiple vitamin B complex, a calcium magnesium vitamin and a vitamin C complex.

For all of you brave-hearted folks who want to go the extra mile, drink one to two tablespoons of apple cider vinegar every morning in ½ cup of water, or mix the vinegar with 1 tablespoon of molasses.

I buy Bragg's Organic Apple Cider Vinegar. Some people mix it with water and drink it that way. Not me! I pour a tall tablespoon and swig it down (*without* holding my nose!). Apple cider vinegar supports friendly-based bacteria. The acids fight against yeast. It also cleanses the digestive system. It is rich in potassium and some research suggests that it will remove calcium deposits from joints and blood vessels and it does not affect the calcium levels in your bones and teeth.

Did you know that Vitamin A keeps your skin beautiful, your eyes healthy and helps prevent infections? Did you know that Vitamin E helps protect Vitamin A and essential fatty acids from cell oxidation? Did you know that Vitamin C helps heal cuts and wounds and keeps teeth and gums healthy? Think of that: you'll never have bad breath. Did you know Vitamin C aids in iron absorption? Wow! Now you know it all!!!

Remember, vitamins are a necessary nutrient that must be obtained either in the diet or by taking supplements. If you have problems with digestion and absorption, you need to eat some raw veggies along with your cooked food. Eating fruits, salads, and raw vegetables will help us get the enzymes our bodies need. It is recommended that we take enzyme caplets because the older we get, the less enzymes we have. We also tend to inhale our food without chewing it, so slow down! Chewing **slowly** is recommended because the chewing process is the beginning of the digestive process. I have included a chart below which lists vitamins and cancer-fighting foods which aid our bodies.

VITAMINS AND CANCER PREVENTION

Vitamin A	Strengthens the immune system. It is essential for mineral metabolism and endocrine function. It helps detoxify our systems. True Vitamin A is found in cod liver oil, fish and shellfish, liver, butter and egg yolks.
Vitamin C	Is an important antioxidant found in many fruits and vegetables.
Vitamins B6 and B12	Deficiencies of these vitamins are associated with cancer and they contribute to the function of over 100 enzymes and are found mostly in animal foods.
Vitamin B17	Protects against cancer and is found in a variety of organically grown grains, legumes, nuts, berries and plants
Vitamin D	Required for mineral absorption and strongly protects against breast and colon cancer.
Vitamin E	Works as an antioxidant and is found in unprocessed oils, nuts (such as almonds) and animal fats like butter and egg yolks.
Conjugated Linoleic Acid	Strongly protects against breast cancer and is found in butter and meat fat.
Cholesterol	A potent antioxidant that protects against free radicals in cell membranes.
Minerals	The body needs generous amounts of zinc, magnesium and selenium. These are vital components of enzymes that help fight carcinogens.
Lactic Acid and Friendly Bacteria	Examples include miso, vinegar-free sauerkraut, citric acid, sugar, keifer and live yogurt cultures and they all contribute to a healthy digestive tract.
Saturated fats	Strengthen the immune system and are needed for proper use of essential fatty acids. The lungs cannot function without saturated fats.
Co-enzyme (Q10)	Highly protective against cancer. Found only in animal foods.

FATS

Fats may be classified as saturated (solid) or unsaturated (liquid). Trans fats are saturated fats which are typically created from unsaturated fats by adding the extra hydrogen atoms in a process called hydrogenation. These are the killers. However, fats or lipids are the most concentrated source of energy in the diet. In addition to providing energy, fats act as carriers for the fat soluble vitamins A, D, E, and K. By aiding in the absorption of vitamin D, fats make calcium available for body tissues, particularly to the bones and teeth. Fats are also important for the conversion of carotene to Vitamin A. There are three essential fatty acids known as linolenic, linoleic, and oleic acids (collectively known as vitamin F). These fatty acids are necessary for normal growth and healthy blood, arteries and nerves. They also keep skin and other tissues youthful and healthy by preventing dry and scaly skin. If you are wondering why your left leg looks like a fish scale, you probably need more Vitamin F. A deficiency of fatty acids may produce eczema and other skin disorders. An extreme deficiency could lead to severely retarded growth. On the other hand, excessive amounts of fat in the diet may lead to abnormal weight gain and obesity if more calories are consumed than are needed by the body. Excessive fat intake will cause abnormally slow digestion and absorption resulting in indigestion. If a lack of carbohydrates is accompanied by a lack of water in the diet or if there is a kidney malfunction, fats cannot be completely metabolized and may become toxic to the body. Soybean oil, safflower oil, canola oil, extra virgin olive oil, castor oil, flax seed oil and fish oil are all good sources of fats. I enjoy cooking with organic, refined expeller pressed safflower oil. This is specifically made for high heat and makes especially yummy (and healthy) fried chicken.

For those of you who enjoy a little fat in your diet, here is some good news. We all need some (good news AND fat, that is!). There are reasons why we have fat pads. These are our cushions. Fat pads aid in reducing or preventing injury to blood vessels, bones, and joints. After a time of fasting, my husband, Richard M., always finds discomfort when he walks around the house because the fat pads on the bottoms of his feet have shrunk. The skin needs fat as it is a provider of elasticity. Adequate fat intake also brings protection from infections. Besides all of that, you need fat on your bones when you are climbing Mt. Everest or skiing in Squaw Valley in the middle

> —∽—
> For those of you who enjoy a little fat in your diet, here is some good news.

of a blizzard. Fat protects our bodies against frigid temperatures. Who knew that fat could protect our toes and fingers from a wicked case of frostbite? The same goes for accidental burns. Long live the fat! P.S. Remember not to take this out of context. We are talking about moderate servings of fat that bring health benefits.

Warning: fat is essential to fertility. A certain percentage of body fat is vital. Women need body fat to ovulate. Studies have shown that 50% of women who have a body mass index (BMI) below 20.7 are infertile. A BMI between 23 and 24 is ideal for conception. The average woman has 20% of her body weight as body fat. Likewise, obesity increases the risk of infertility. Extra fat produces extra estrogen in the system, causing an imbalance in the ratio of the reproductive hormones needed for an egg to release and ripen. Here is the really good news. The effect can be quickly reversed. Just losing a small amount of weight will be enough to stimulate regular ovulation.

CARBOHYDRATES

Carbohydrates are the chief source of energy for brain power, body functions, and muscular exertion and they assist in the digestion and assimilation of other foods. Carbohydrates also help regulate protein and fat metabolism. Fats require carbohydrates for their breakdown within the liver. The principal carbohydrates present in foods are sugars, starches, and cellulose and there are two types: simple carbohydrates and complex carbohydrates. The difference is important to nutrition because complex carbohydrates take longer to metabolize and simple carbohydrates are metabolized quickly, thus raising blood sugar levels more quickly and causing rapid increases in blood insulin levels.

> ## The key here, again, is to find a balance.

All sugars and starches are converted by the digestive juices to a simple sugar called glucose. This glucose, or blood sugar, is used as fuel by tissues of the brain, nervous system and muscles. A small portion of the glucose is converted to glycogen and stored by the liver and muscles. The excess is then converted to fat and stored throughout the body as a reserved source of energy. When fat reserves are reconverted to glucose and used for fuel, weight loss occurs. Carbohydrate snacks containing sugars and starches provide the body with instant energy because they cause a sudden rise in the blood sugar level. However, the blood sugar level then drops again rapidly, creating a craving for more sweet foods, and in its aftermath, can cause fatigue, dizziness, nervousness, and headaches. Foods such as white flour, white sugar, and polished or white rice are lacking in B vitamin nutrients. If B vitamins are absent, carbohydrate combustion cannot take place. Instead, heartburn, indigestion, and nausea may result. Please note that B vitamins should be taken in a balanced B complex, so check the label to ensure that this is the case. Additionally, if you take B12 shots, ask the doctor to give you half B12 and half complex in order to stay balanced. Research suggests that diabetes, heart disease, high blood pressure, anemia, kidney disorders, and cancer may be linked to an overabundant consumption of carbohydrate foods in a diet. On the flip side, a lack of carbohydrates may produce ketosis, loss of energy, depression, and a breakdown of essential body proteins. The key here, again, is to find a balance.

We must also be careful about popular fad diets because these can cause dangerous induction periods during massive protein intake. The omission of carbohydrates can cause serious health problems such as kidney impairment. Carbohydrates are fuel for the body and they are not bad when consumed in moderation. Remember that even Jesus ate bread at the Passover. Recall the story of the *loaves* and the fishes (not rib eye steaks and fishes) and receive the go-ahead from me to consume carbohydrates. Complex carbohydrates are a much better choice than simple carbohydrates and the key is to eat them in moderation. The following quotation, "Everything too much is not good for you," is worth repeating to yourself every day. Complex carbohydrates are found in foods such as whole wheat bread with fiber. They last longer, make you feel satisfied longer, and as a rule are much more beneficial than the simple carbohydrates found in white bread and rice, which both contain bleaching agents. Healthy choices are better choices!

PROTEINS

Proteins are the structural materials of our muscle, skin, and hair. Sources of protein include meat, eggs, fish, soy products, grains, and legumes (which include alfalfa, clover, peas, beans, lentils, and peanuts). Dairy products such as milk and cheese are also great sources of protein. Lean choices of meat include loin, round and leg. Remember to trim the fat and remove skin before or after cooking meats. We need approximately one gram of protein per kilogram of body mass which is about the size of the palm of our hand. Athletes who play power sports typically require approximately two grams of protein per day for each kilogram of body weight. This is double the amount required by a sedentary person. We need to eat the proper amount of protein in order to maintain good health. It is also critical that we not overload on protein as we then run the risk of stressing out our vital organs. We see so much of this in the high protein fad diets which require an overabundance of proteins and a minimum amount of carbohydrates. Our bodies require a balance of proteins and carbohydrates in order to eliminate fats and waste. Proteins are necessary for the regulation of nearly everything that happens in our bodies and carbohydrates give us energy and allow our brains to function at full capacity.

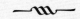

> Our bodies require a balance of proteins and carbohydrates in order to eliminate fats and waste.

MINERALS

Minerals are essential for our daily nutritional balance. Although only 4 or 5 percent of our body weight is made up of mineral matter, minerals are vital to our overall mental and physical well being. Bones, teeth, soft tissue, muscles, blood, and nerve cells are made up of minerals. They are also important factors in maintaining psychological processes such as perception, sensation, learning and memory, cognition, and the processing of information. Minerals strengthen our skeletal structures and preserve the vigor of our hearts, brains, muscles and nervous systems. The two types of minerals are macro and trace minerals. Macro minerals are present in large amounts of our body tissue and consist of calcium chloride, magnesium phosphorous, potassium, sodium and sulfur. Trace minerals exist in minute quantities and are essential to proper body functioning. These include cobalt, copper, chromium, iodine, iron, manganese, molyedenum, nickel selenium, vanadium, and zinc. I realize that this may sound like a foreign language, but simply put, a balanced diet of meats and vegetables will help fulfill your daily mineral requirements.

FIBER

Fruits and vegetables are the Mercedes Benz of fiber. Since some of you do not understand the importance of including fiber in your diet, let me put on a light show for you. Imagine a parade with floats where people are carrying the bull horn and red flags and shouting the words, "EAT FIBER!!!" This is the stuff that provides bulk to the intestinal contents (don't pretend you don't know what I'm talking about). It promotes peristalsis, a wavelike motion that pushes food downward. This is a touchy subject. Lack of fiber leads to constipation which may leave you feeling like a cement truck that has been sitting in the sun for three days. This is serious business. Constipation can cause some horrific intestinal pain and embarrassing, gassy moments. Trust me. This is tough on relationships, especially if it is your very first date. It also causes agonizing problems such as bowel obstruction, colonic diseases, cancer, polyps, hemorrhoids, diverticulitis, bloating, gas (YIKES!!), cramps, headaches, dizziness, insomnia, discomfort and even re-absorption of toxic wastes. In order to ensure that you are getting enough fiber, you need to eat five servings of fruits and vegetables per day. You really should be eating fiber during every meal. If you are not currently getting enough fiber in your diet, there are many sources of fiber you can buy. Read the packages at the grocery store and pick out items that contain high amounts of fiber. Please also look for items that do not contain aspartame or other artificial sweeteners as these hinder the digestive process.

Fiber also helps us lose weight. Foods that are high in fiber are usually low in fat and calories, so we are eating healthier just by eating fiber-rich foods. I used to watch Old Daisy the cow chew her oats and her alfalfa. I marveled back then that it seemed to take Daisy an eternity to eat her mid-morning snack, but I now understand that foods rich in fiber take longer to chew, so again, we need to eat slower. Savor the flavor! We will get full faster and it will last longer. My doctor constantly reminds me that fiber may prevent or reduce the risk of developing cancer, diabetes, and also may reduce the risk of heart disease by lowering LDL (or bad) cholesterol.

THE BENEFITS OF WATER

We seem to be in a great deficit for clear and pure drinking water in our world and we need to understand and appreciate the benefit of pure water. When we drink water, the cells in our faces are hydrated. The whites of our eyes become whiter. Collapsed veins are revived. We lose weight when we drink water. Even fetuses depend on water. They are surrounded by it for nine months because it protects them. "Drinking lots and lots of water is wonderful for the skin," says Marrianne O'Donohue, M.D., Associate Professor of Dermatology at Rush Presbyterian-St. Luke's Medical Center. The skin needs water to maintain its correct internal temperature and water keeps the body flushed.

For you complainers who say that you hate to drink water, here is your answer: there are many variations of water such as tap water, bottled water, still water, sparkling water, flavored water (still and sparkling) and you can also buy those little flavored powder packets, dump them into your bottle of water, shake it up and drink it down. Just stop the complaining and drink it. We need eight glasses per day and the benefits are priceless.

Americans drank more than 8.2 billion gallons of bottled water in 2006. That equals 28 gallons per person, or half a gallon per week. Americans drink more bottled water than milk, coffee or beer (hopefully you don't drink beer at all!) I understand that buying bottled water can be expensive, so please note that the water which comes out of your kitchen sink routinely wins taste tests over bottled water and costs a tiny fraction of the $1.64 per gallon that Americans spend on the bottled stuff, according to ACNielsen, an international market research firm based in Illinois.

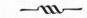

The water which comes out of your kitchen sink routinely wins taste tests over bottled water.

Here are some easy ways to wet your whistle. Always keep a fresh pitcher of water on your nightstand and on your desk at work. Use a 12 to 16 oz. tumbler so that you will only have to drink 4 to 6 glasses each day. I also try to find interesting looking water containers for my family because my grandchildren love to carry water thermoses with cool designs. One easy and healthy change I have made is that in the morning, instead of drinking a cup of coffee or tea, I drink a cup of hot water with lemon slices.

7

metabolism and Exercise

GET MOVING!!! Appropriate exercise will help you get going. I used to be a jogger, but as I crossed that Great Divide of 50 years old, I decided to instead consider the longevity of my joints and sockets. There are other factors to consider for boosting a sluggish metabolism. Green tea is a wonderful kick start for your metabolism. A health professional told me that we die when we do not move and we die when we do not breathe. If you prefer less movement and less oxygen, then get yourself ready for the walker, the wheelchair, and the retirement community. Otherwise, get yourself filled up on oxygen and have the go-get-em' spirit. You will be tearing it up as an octogenarian. So breathe, breathe, breathe and move, move, move!

Have you ever heard of mitochondria? This is a cellular process that combines the calories you consume with oxygen and then turns this combination into energy which is used to run your entire body. The rate at which your mitochondria transform food and oxygen into energy is called your metabolic rate. This is determined by two factors. The first is the number of mitochondria you have and the second is how efficiently they burn oxygen and calories. The more mitochondria you have, the more efficiently they consume oxygen and the faster your metabolic rate, the easier it is for your body to burn calories and the more energy you will have. That was definitely a run-on sentence, but I'm leaving it in. Here it is again: EXERCISE! When you exercise you increase muscle mass and you increase oxygen intake. By increasing your muscle mass, you increase the number of cells in your body that contain large amounts of mitochondria. Your muscles have the highest concentration of mitochondria. Exercise increases your metabolic power. This is incredible because it affects not only the number of calories you burn during exercise, but also the calories you burn when you are not exercising. By increasing the number and function of the mitochondria in your body, you increase your ability to burn calories at rest. Imagine burning calories when you are taking a nap!

Imagine burning calories when you are taking a nap!

Our son Richard, currently studying in pre-med, motivates us to exercise consistently and live an active lifestyle. He told us that regular exercise massages the muscles and organs. It literally sweeps through the lymph glands, washing away mucous poisons and purifying our systems. Exercise is any exertion that is performed to improve health, shape or performance. It can help you lose weight, strengthen your heart and lungs, increase bone density, give you more energy, help you sleep better, reduce stress, enhance your mood, relieve symptoms of depression and anxiety and even reduce the risk of heart disease and certain types of cancer. Any exercise is beneficial to your physical and mental health.

One of the preferred benefits of exercising is weight loss. Sometimes we exercise just because we love to sweat, and sometimes we want to run the race and win. When we exercise, it sends endorphins which reduce our stress levels and the good Lord knows that most of us are on overload right now. Another great reason to exercise is that we will live longer and feel younger. Exercising adds years to your life. Barring any unforeseen circumstances, men who exercise on a consistent basis can add possibly eight years to their life span and women can add possibly nine years.

Getting your heart to beat at its maximum and breaking a sweat has long term benefits. Up to twelve hours after you have exercised, your metabolism is still working to burn up excess calories. This means that even after you have eaten a meal (not including two loaves of French bread and a pound of butter with a piece of Godiva chocolate cheesecake) your body will continue to rid itself of the extra calories. It is essential that you increase your heart rate for at least 20 minutes as you exercise. The following chart, taken from my own treadmill, shows the appropriate rate at which our hearts should beat per minute during exercise for each age bracket. Again, please make sure that you get a physical and consult with your physician before starting a regimented exercise program.

0 yrs.	25 yrs.	30 yrs.	35 yrs.	40 yrs.	45 yrs.	50 yrs.	55 yrs.	60 yrs.	65 yrs.
70	166	162	157	153	149	145	140	136	132

There is a huge list of exercise programs. Pick one and stick with it. Consistency is the key. Get inspired. Do not get locked into an unrealistic exercise program that you hate. This should be your time to regenerate. Use this time to change the way you live, the way you breathe, and your outlook on life. You are doing something good for your body in order to become everything you need to be for God and for the people who love and need you.

Before I jump back onto my exercise soapbox, let me talk to you for a moment about the importance of proper breathing. Breathing is something that most of us take for granted. It is an involuntary action that requires no thought, so why talk about it? Well, let me answer that question. Besides the fact that it is an essential action required for us to continue walking this earth, it is also a powerful oxygen-delivering action that, when practiced properly, will soothe nerves and bring calm to a stressful day. With high blood pressure and stress levels flying through the roof, we need to step back one to two minutes each day and practice some breathing exercises. I promise it will not take a long time and it is 100% free. Why don't we give it a go right now! Ready?

1. **Lengthen your body**: Sit or stand, with both feet flat on the floor. Imagine the top of your head extending toward the ceiling. This creates space in the spine and torso and allows your lungs to expand fully.

2. **Inhale:** Take a deep, full breath. Picture your abdomen filling with air from the bottom of your belly. Then, picture your lungs filling with air to the top of your chest. This brings oxygen into your cells which restores and energizes your whole body.

3. **Exhale:** Blow out your breath and imagine it coming out from the top of the lungs to the lowest part of the belly. At the same time, mentally let go of anything that is bothering you. The exhalation of air detoxifies your body. Simply put, this is just a loooooong "sigh" which works to release as much emotional energy as it does air.

4. **Pause:** When you reach the end of your exhale, rest for a moment before you inhale again, without tightening or holding your breath. Repeat this once or twice and just relax for a moment. This creates a moment of stillness that will help slow your mind down and relax your body.

In addition to helping us calm down and alleviating outside stressors, breathing properly is also key during exercise. For example, when exercising, remember to breathe in your nose, out your mouth, in your nose, out your mouth, etc. If you do not discipline yourself to breathe properly, you may end up hyperventilating and falling off your treadmill.

Let's talk about breathing in the good air and releasing the bad air. Just a few nights ago, our oldest daughter, Mindy, gave birth to her twin girls, Sophia and Isabella. They are extraordinarily beautiful babies. (Listen to the old crow!). These little ones are blessed to have Gilbert and Mindy as their parents and I am quite sure they will adore their two handsome older brothers, Taylor and Josiah. Now, the birth of the twins was quite an event. The labor room was filled with family, church family and friends. I am sure the nurses were not too happy with us and would have liked to shut down the party. It looked and smelled like a florist shop. Everywhere were beautiful bouquets, balloons and lattes. I observed the room and thought,

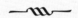

I cried when the first baby came and cried again when the second little one was born.

"Wow! Do we know how to have babies or what?!" Gilbert could most definitely get a side job as a labor coach. At the beginning and end of each contraction, he encouraged Mindy to take a deep cleansing breath and then to release the tension and relax every part of her body. There were times when the contractions were so painful and he had to remind her, "Breathe now, baby. That's good. Okay. You're doing great." I watched the monitors as they registered the babies' heartbeats. Mindy was laboring hard but remained constantly aware of how important it was to bring clean, fresh oxygen to her little girls. I cried when the first baby came and cried again when the second little one was born. She was breech and came out feet first. Mindy was unbelievable and breathed strongly throughout the entire delivery.

As we take in our daily dosage of oxygen, we should also be conscious of the way we are breathing in and out. When we inhale, we should breathe in new energy, life, love, joy, peace and contentment. When we exhale we should release every negative hurt along with anything that takes away our energy. As our lungs expand, we must fill them with air and then slowly release the air and repeat this several times. Be sure and take all of the time you need and do not ever force your breaths.

> When we inhale, we should breathe in new energy, life, love, joy, peace and contentment.

If you feel like a nervous wreck and are having a beastly, exasperating moment, please try this simple breathing exercise. Find a comfortable position and relax your whole body. Your hands should be still in your lap. Do not fold your arms or legs. Close your eyes. Now breathe. Try to count to seven as you breathe in. Now, breathe out and count to seven again. When you finish, your frayed nerves should be considerably calmed down. If you still feel edgy or jittery, repeat this exercise as needed.

I would be a millionaire if I could get back all of the money I have spent signing up for exercise programs only to go three times and quit. It was too much of an effort for me to get dressed, drive to class, and spend excess time on the freeway. So, I purchased my treadmill, put it in my garage and I am painfully struggling, striving and endeavoring to jog or speed walk at least two miles a day, three times per week.

As an alternative to just walking on the treadmill at the same speed, the exercise gurus recommend a 35 minute workout on the treadmill that will increase your heart rate. I alternate between walking 5 minutes at a clipped speed. Then, I walk or jog 3 to 4 minutes on the fastest speed that I can. I repeat this process for the entire duration of my workout. Typically, I can walk or jog 3 miles in 35 minutes. I finish my workout with a slower pace which allows me to cool down and gives my heart the chance to return to its normal pulse. **It is critically important that you allow time for your body to warm up at the beginning of your workout. It is equally important that you allow your body time to cool down at the end of your workout.**

Along with walking or jogging, my daughter, Kate, has taught me some Pilates stretches which are great at conditioning, lengthening and keeping muscles limber. Kate has also added to my routine a series of weight training with five pound weights. As we age, it is important to do some sort of weight resistance.

If you have not moved a muscle in 35 years, please take it REALLY easy. Start with the non-threatening stuff. Do not go for the 40 pound dumbbell. Although it is a known fact that there are great benefits to weight training, please start with five pound weights and work your way up as your body becomes conditioned to the weights. Weight training adds lean muscle mass to your body which will consume more calories than fat which helps to keep your weight down. Muscles add durability and strength and yes, the good news is that as you exercise and strengthen your lower back muscles you will say good bye to lower back pain. Exercising also makes your heart, arteries and immune system younger. But most of all, using weights literally fills up our bones. It is one of the best things for maintaining and building bone density along with preventing osteoporosis. Here is an amazing fact. Bone forms in our bodies in response to stress! Now, here is the deal. You do not have to bench press or lift a sack of 100 pound beans. Just do some resistance training such as aquatic aerobics. The water adds an incredible amount of resistance and burns tons of calories. Swimming is not only fun. In my opinion, it is also the easiest and safest way to fulfill your resistance exercise.

Some additional resistance exercises you can do are lunges or squats. These are great to start with. Crunches work your mid-section and are extremely strength-building exercises. Millions of Americans have extreme back pain and much of this could be alleviated by strengthening the abdominal and pelvic muscles. Do 10 to 30 minute intervals three times per week to keep that muscle mass where it needs to be. There will be a consequence in later years if you are not committed right now to stay consistent. Please remember that we lose 5% of our muscle mass every 10 years. If we choose not to take a few minutes every day to do these exercises, there is a strong possibility that we will turn into a Gumby look-alike.

Ninety-three-year-old Reverend Norman Milbank is the principal of Canterbury Christian School where my children attended and now my grandchildren attend and he is committed to his daily exercise. He lifts weights and swims against the current in his wave pool every day. This has bought him great quality of life as he develops and mentors others. He is a constant inspiration to those around him as he continually imparts his wisdom and passion for life. He is strong both physically and mentally because of the many years of his tenacious discipline. I am confident that he will still be lecturing and ministering to parents and their children long after he has crossed the 100 year mark. When I am tempted to skip my daily routine, I think of Reverend Milbank and I go put my tennis shoes on and start moving immediately.

8

emotional Wellness

Anger, Depression, Forgiveness and Peace

A nger is the strongest and most forceful emotion we experience. It is undoubtedly the least useful and most devastating. Unharnessed anger destroys relationships and eventually ruins our health. Hopefully you have figured out by now that the reason I am including a section on anger is due to my concern for our emotional wellness.

I have seen what anger does to families. It is equal to a hurricane in its destruction. Just one family member raging with anger can produce a torrent of crippling emotions that leave the rest of the family dealing with insecurity, fear, frustration, depression, and an overall dysfunction that ultimately limits the depth and strength of all other relationships. A study was released by scientists and psychologists who cited the consistent deterioration of the immune system when it is constantly assaulted by negative emotions. Anger is not only abusive to the recipient, but it is equally hurtful to the one who is filled with anger. There are two levels of angry people. Type I is the angry hothead. People walk on eggshells around the angry hothead, hoping and praying that they will not do or say anything to trigger any feelings of anger in this person. Type II is the angry *internal* hothead who hides or suppresses their emotions. They control their outward anger to the extent that most people have absolutely no clue that these emotions are raging inside this person. Be advised that when you suppress raw anger, your unfortunate stomach keeps the score. To be angry and never show it is even more detrimental to your health and your emotional well being. Type I is destructive to people around them and Type II is more destructive to themselves. To quote a dear friend of mine, Leanne Kimmell, "Anger is like drinking poison and expecting it to kill someone else." If you are a Type II person, please understand you are only hurting and destroying yourself and your good life. You can tell a lot about an angry personality by three things: how often they get angry, the relative importance of the things that anger them, and how long they stay angry.

We need to deal with our anger for many reasons. Anger ruins our relationships and our happiness. Individuals who harbor anger toward others are more likely to die of heart disease and are also more likely to die prematurely. Let's face it. When we are full of anger we say, do, and feel things we should not say, do, or feel. A friend once confessed to me that when she gets mad, she goes directly to McDonald's and orders everything she wants, including a double cheeseburger, large fries and a large Coke. She also admitted that these actions only add to her frustration and anger and make her feel perpetually grumpy. If you want MY true confession, I was so angry one night that I went fast food hopping. I went to four fast food joints and then finished off my rampage with Krispy Kreme donuts at midnight. The next morning I could barely peel myself off of my sheets. My stomach was cemented to my bed.

I am speaking not from book knowledge, but from real experience. Anger will wear us down emotionally, physically and spiritually and can cause major meltdown and burnout. When we live in anger, it keeps us from living a Wholly Fit life. Angry people have trouble living according to Galatians 5:22-24 which states, "But the fruit of the spirit is love, joy, peace, longsuffering, gentleness, goodness, faith, meekness, temperance, against such there is no law and they that are in Christ have crucified the flesh…if we live in the spirit, let us also walk in the spirit." In other words, if we claim to be people of the spirit, then we also need to practice self-control or temperance.

You cannot be an angry-spirited person and simultaneously display the fruits of the spirit in your life. Anger causes conflict in the lives of others. Proverbs 15:18 says, "A wrathful man stirs up strife, but he that is slow to anger appeases strife." When you are angry, it is contagious and causes others to become angry as well. Proverbs 22:24-25 goes on to tell us, "Make no friendship with a man given to anger nor go with a wrathful man lest you learn his ways and entangle yourself in a snare" (English Standard Version). If you associate with angry people, there is a great possibility that you will become like them and take on their angry nature. The old adage is true. Birds of a feather do flock together! Children who grow up in angry environments usually express traits of anger and most often become angry spouses and produce angry children. There is always the exception to the rule, however. You can **choose** a better way to live. An angry father brings trouble to his family. He destroys the integrity he should bring to his wife and children. Proverbs 29:11 tells us "A fool utters his entire mind, but a wise man keeps it until afterwards." In other words, chill out, think about it and *then* speak your piece. The

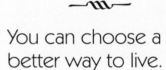

You can choose a better way to live.

worst possible thing we can do is to give someone a piece of our mind!!!!!!!!!!!!!! Why should we give our mind away when we have so little to begin with?

The story of King Saul underscores the importance of living an anger-free life. David was becoming popular among his people. This angered King Saul. Someone had written a new song which quickly climbed the charts until it reached #1 on the play list. The hook of the song was this: "Saul has slain his thousands, but David has slain his ten thousands…" Saul became full of wrath and was extremely displeased with what the people were saying. He was enraged with jealousy and hostile anger and he put the evil eye on David from that day forward. Unfortunately for King Saul, he allowed himself to be overtaken by anger and he ultimately lost his integrity and later lost his entire kingdom to David.

When we *allow* other people to stir up hostility and anger in us, we must realize that we are also giving away our kingdom. We give up our health, our peace of mind and our contentment. That's right. That is *exactly* what I said. We GIVE it away. I know people who over and over again have let anger destroy them from the inside out. Please remember this. Other people cannot take our peace, happiness, contentment or joy. **We** are the ones who give them away. We give up our rights and entitlement to the good things God has intended for us to enjoy, including a body that functions correctly and works to its fullest potential. Here is a little food for thought. There will always be somebody who is better than you, and who is more talented and gifted than you. There will also be someone with more money, greater influence and more importance than you, so you might as well relax, do your best at whatever you are doing and enjoy the journey. Leave the rest up to the Lord. It is what He thinks that actually counts, after all. If you truly want to be a strong leader and a person of influence, you must wholeheartedly refrain from giving yourself over to a wrathful or angry spirit. Titus 1:7, in the middle of the verse tells us to be "…not soon angry…" In other words, don't blow your cool, man!

Dr. S.I. McMillan's basic idea in his book, *None of These Diseases,* was that most physical problems stem from emotional upsets. Over 70% of patients in the hospital are suffering from something that began as an emotional upheaval. He wrote, "The moment I start hating a man, I become his slave. I cannot enjoy my work anymore because he controls my thoughts. My resentment towards a man produces too many stress hormones in my body and eventually I become fried after a few hours of work. The work that I formally enjoyed becomes a drudgery. Even vacations will not bring me pleasure because the man I hate goes with me wherever I go. I cannot escape his grasp upon my mind."

A dear friend of mine was diagnosed with multiple sclerosis (MS) and has suffered for years with this dreadful illness. He has been a man of great faith and he continually thanked God in anticipation of the physical healing he so desperately desired. He was militant about eating the appropriate foods and getting the proper amounts of exercise and rest. He believed in divine healing as the scripture teaches and throughout his Christian life, he was prayed for many times. Even though he believed God had healed him, the MS symptoms returned over and over again, until one day a minister spoke a word of knowledge into his life. The minister was impressed by the Spirit of God to tell him that the reason he was never able to receive complete healing was because as a small child he had suffered terrible sexual abuse and had never been able to deal with it. At the very moment the minister spoke this revelation, the man was instantly and completely healed, both emotionally and physically. Only when we make the decision to release our hurt and pain will we truly receive help, healing and wholeness through the delivering power of Jesus' name. I also recommend resolution of internal conflict through the wisdom of spirit-filled counselors who can help us see outside ourselves.

There are eight causes of anger with fear being #1 in line and leading the rest of the pack. We all know what it feels like to be frightened. When a car swerves all over the road, crosses the line and heads straight toward us, we experience fear in the *raw*, mixed with anger.

Frustration. Have you ever dealt with a stubborn 2-year-old or 14-year old? Need I say more? If you are unsure about the definition of frustration, you need to go read about Moses and his extended family in Exodus. Most of the time, those unhappy children of Israel were grumbling and complaining about everything. Moses finally lost it. He pushed the anger envelope by striking the rock two times. The water indeed came out, but so did his wrath. Because of his disobedience (brought on by uncontrolled anger) Moses was not able to cross over into the Promised Land.

Violation of rights. We become angry when we think people are violating the rights that we deserve. We also become angry if we feel that people are getting into our space.

Disappointment. We feel that we have missed out. We look back over the years we have lived and then we look at our current station in life. We wonder why we have not accomplished what we had so carefully planned out and earnestly desired for ourselves.

Misunderstood. We have ALL been here. We feel like screaming, "Wait a minute! This is not fair!! It's not right! You don't know the whole story. If you knew the whole story from A to Z, you would NOT say those things about me!" Henry Beret says, "Other people don't create your spirit. They only reveal it." I also hear this statement so often, "They made me sooooooo mad!" To which my response is, "No. They just pushed your angry buttons and your weakness was revealed!" Let it go. It is just not worth the defensive argument to prove to someone that they have wronged you. Be the bigger person and walk away.

Mistrust. There is a definite connection between mistrusting people and an angry spirit. Interestingly, people who trust other people typically have very little anger issues. Hey! Open your heart up a tad! Be vulnerable. You may surprise yourself at the pleasant feelings you begin to have toward other people!

Unrealistic expectations. I was completely set free the day I learned about unrealistic expectations. I was reborn! We become angry when we have high expectations of what we think other people should do or be. Simply put, we need to anticipate without the unrealistic expectations. We also need to give ourselves and others some slack.

Bitterness. This is the deepest root of all anger. Please, my dear friends, let me speak into your life right now. If you are bitter, you have a true heart disease going on which will affect your life in every possible way. I am talking about spiritually, emotionally, physically and mentally. Hebrews 12:15 says, "Looking diligently lest any man fail of the grace of God." (lest any root of bitterness springing up troubles you and thereby a man be defiled).

Now that you have been provided you with the eight causes of anger, here is a checklist to help you assess any negative emotions that could possibly reveal hidden anger issues.

Is my anger cruel to others? Check out the story of Joseph in Genesis 50. Joseph epitomized grace while his long-lost sinner brothers were the poster children for wickedness. Grace usually has the last word in family feuds as it did in Joseph's family when he said, "I know you guys left me freezing and starving and you hoped I would end up as bear bait and coyote canapés appetizers, but God had other plans. He had a big banquet prepared just for me!" Actually, the literal Word says, "I know you meant it for evil, but God meant it for good." I happen to think Joseph successfully avoided suffering from acid reflux, gall bladder trouble and anxiety-induced shingles because he absolutely refused to keep score of the hurt and backstabbing (not to *mention* the underhanded, out of control, ego-eating, and jealousy-belching wickedness). None of these things were able to choke out the goodness of God's righteousness. Joseph *refused* to be angry at his brothers. As my wise, dear friend, D. Harris (long-time CIA agent turned missionary/mentor/marvelous mother in Israel) says, "Just grace it!"

Does my anger cause me to lose my temper? Proverbs 12:16 tells us that a fool's anger is known at once.

Does my anger stir up others? The problem with anger is that it is a contagious emotion. It affects others around it as it spreads.

Does my anger intimidate others? If Elijah were alive today, I would ask him about Jezebel and her Jeopardy moments. I am sure he would shed some serious light on this subject. One minute the prophet Elijah was totally uninhibited. He displayed great power and confidence as he called down fire from Heaven and torched those false prophets until they were toast. He left the entire top of Mt. Carmel looking like it had been nuked. A little later in the story, though, he was terrified and running for his life. That's right. Our hero, Elijah, was ready to call it quits and join that great and mighty cloud of witnesses. Intimidation is real! If you use your angry face to scare people, I hope you wake up in the morning to find frogs in your toilet and lizards in your tub…or… well…I suppose you may think I am being a bit over-dramatic here, but please understand that anger which engages intimidation is evil. STOP IT!!!!!!!!!! Do NOT allow it to rear its ugly head again. Say, "I promise!!"

Could my anger lead to harming others? Richard M. and I have counseled many people over the years who have confessed to living with painful memories of horrible things they did and abusive words they spoke to others. The unfortunate consequence is that they now live in constant regret. If they had kept their anger in check many years ago, the terribly abusive words and physical harm inflicted on others might have been avoided. We must be accountable in this area to someone we trust and we must put a limit on our anger.

Does my anger cause me to seek revenge against others? It is not up to us to settle the score. It is God who sees the beginning from the end. He is a just and sovereign God and we must give Him full control of not only our emotions, but our whole lives as well. Nothing good will come out of seeking our own revenge. We must leave it alone and recite the scripture (over and over if it helps!) "Vengeance is mine sayeth the Lord and I will repay…" We must let God fix it. He is the best "fixer" I know.

Does my anger show a lack of Godly love? In I Corinthians 13:5 the Apostle Paul chiseled away at careless attitudes that screamed, "I could 'care less' what they think or how they feel. They can get over it!!!" Paul tells us that when we are filled with the attributes of Christ's love, we are infused with love and ultimately, we become love. We will not, do not and cannot act unbecomingly. In other words, we will not be consumed with anger.

As you complete the above evaluation on yourself, be honest. Are you prone to sudden outbursts? Do people put on their kid gloves and walk on eggshells when they are with you? Are you high maintenance? Can people truly relax and be themselves around you? If you are brutally honest, you may see some things about yourself that you really need to work on. I took the test and OUCH, I discovered some things in my own life that needed to be worked on. That hurt!

When dealing with our anger, we must remember to deal with it in a proper manner. We must not nurse, disperse or rehearse our anger. All three of these responses to anger are wrong.

NURSING OUR ANGER

Humans have a natural tendency to hide behind anger. Ephesians 4:26-27 says, "Do not let the sun go down on your wrath..." In other words, do not hide it. Do not feed it. Do not pretend that it is not there. Just fix it! Many times the terrible and dreaded disease, cancer, will seed itself and begin cell multiplication in our bodies. It then becomes a deadly, voracious monster as tumors begin to spread and then mastisize into other vulnerable, unsuspecting areas. The CAT scan shows absolutely nothing. The x-rays are clear. The ultrasound is normal and yet the blood tells a different story. Beyond the shadow of a doubt, something is wrong, yet it is hard to pinpoint the where and what. When we hide our anger, it multiplies, grows and spreads. We must NOT let it spread. We must deal with it and make it right before we let another moment pass. A research study concluded that women who repress and refuse to deal with their anger are three times more likely to die at an earlier age than those who are able to express anger in a productive manner. I suggest that we immediately deal with our anger.

DISPERSING OUR ANGER

This is an accident waiting to happen and it will show up in many areas of our lives. I have spent time with people who can completely take the joy out of the most incredible vacations. Everything is intense and nothing is right as these people draw lines and keep score cards on things that simply do not matter! A casual lunch turns into a bloody battlefield and everyone who interacts with this angry person is pumped full of shrapnel and ready to meet the paramedics. As a matter of fact, marriage for this type of person is a battlefield. Their family is a battlefield. Their work place is a battlefield. Their entire LIFE is a battlefield. You had better bring the helicopter, the stretchers, and the oxygen. Ephesians 4:29-30 says, "...Let no corrupt communication proceed out of your mouth." Corrupt in the Greek origin means "cutting." Do not allow anything to come out of your mouth that will cut people down and hurt them. This is the result of unresolved anger. This is the bedfellow of unabbreviated bitterness. Anger equals a cutting word, a bitter word, and a jealous word. Okay, all that talk about anger is such a downer. I want to talk about edification.

To edify means to build up and is the complete opposite of corrupt, which means to tear down. When we choose to edify, we minister grace unto the hearers. When we choose to tear people down, we give ourselves over to an angry, jealous spirit. Ephesians 4:30 says, "…And grieve not the Holy Spirit of God…" Corrupt communication grieves the Spirit of God and we can avoid grieving the Spirit of God by edifying and building up people. This idea

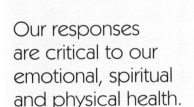

Our responses are critical to our emotional, spiritual and physical health.

makes the Lord smile on us. Plus, our responses are critical to our emotional, spiritual and physical health.

REHEARSING OUR ANGER

When I was a child, I was encouraged to practice the piano and I practiced *diligently* every day. There are selected classical pieces that I practiced many times and that I still find myself trying to master today. Just as I have sought to master the art of classical music, there are people (poor souls) such as the vagabonds, the homeless, the threadbare, and the naked-in-spirit kind of people I have been acquainted with who have resolved themselves to spending their lifetime mastering their bitter monologues. They want everyone to know how badly they have been treated and how terrible life has been to them. You know who I am talking about. These are the Bad News Bettys of life, the Bitter Beckys who live to take other people down, and the Hateful Harriets who blow their green, putrid stink of death in your face. Oh, and one more thing: everything bad that has ever happened to them is your fault. You are the sole reason they cannot have a good life. You are the one who created all the bad breaks in their life. Because of you, their life is tough. You derailed their dreams. You stole their happiness. Whoa, whoa,

whoa! Hang on just a second. How much more do you want to take? Now, I know we are supposed to love everyone (we do) and I know we are encouraged to help everybody (we do!). We should be good listeners, compassionate givers, and sincere in our tender care for all people, but we must draw a line somewhere! We have to set boundaries that other people cannot cross. At some point we have to say, "ENOUGH!!!"

These individuals need to take responsibility for their own lives *right* here and *right* now. They must make the choice to get over it and move on. This goes for you too. If you are sweating right now and feeling your pulse quicken, my guess is that you are more than familiar with some (or all) of these characteristics. Take a truth test and just admit that you stink. Your spouse, children, friends, dogs, cats and chickens will appreciate you so much more for your forthright honesty. You may even win the high achievement award for Most Improved Person of the Year. If you are not the one struggling with the anger problem, but the person you live with or your co-worker is struggling, stop being passive aggressive and pretending that everything is hunky dory. Because we feel intimated by angry people, it is never an easy task to confront them. However, let me give you some advice so we can get this show on the road. Do it anyway! Confront the person immediately and acknowledge their anger. Tell them you understand that they are angry. It is important that they know you are concerned about their anger and that you have a sincere attitude. Tell them you feel badly that they are terribly upset. Then listen to them even though it may take a few minutes of your time. Eventually they will run out of steam. (Actually, it may take months or even a lifetime. My dad is going to be 80 years old soon and he is still running on a full tank of steam, but don't let that discourage you).

> We have to set boundaries that other people cannot cross.

Angry people have to vent, so let them. Do not try to defend yourself. This only stirs them up further and keeps them in an uproar. Stay calm. I know this is not easy to do, but it is ever sooooo empowering. In our humanity we want to defend ourselves and respond with, "What do you mean I'm difficult? I cannot understand why you would be angry with me!" When someone is raking me over the burning hot coals I just tell myself repeatedly that in 77 years it will not matter anyway. Why sweat the small stuff? Why let this person's problem destroy my peace? I can refuse to let them. If they insist on self-destruction then I can only hope and pray they do not succeed. I choose to rise above their deathly entrapment of angry bitterness. It is their prison, not mine.

Next, try to remember that most often there is something else underneath the surface of their anger. Angry people have unresolved issues in their lives which they have never brought to a place of closure. Instead, these things have lain dormant for many years because the person has not found the strength or courage to deal with the painful memories once and for all. They have never been able to truly let the situation go. Has someone who is madder than a wet hen ever blown up at you? If so, you will eventually find out that it had nothing to do with you at all! It was the clanking of a scary, silent skeleton resurrected from their entombed, hurtful memories of a long, long, long time ago.

Make a decision. For your own peace of mind, you must both come to an agreement of when the problem will be fixed. It is human tendency to appease the person who is angry. We just want to placate their feelings and let it slide. However, we can NOT do that. Here is the kicker. If angry people are not confronted with a time table to fix the problem, they become even angrier. In fact, the process of unabated anger goes something like this: the angry person begins to run over us and at some point they may even become physically abusive. The tendency is to back off and not do anything because we think their anger will subside. Please be advised that more often than not, it will NOT subside. You are not the reason the anger started in the first place and it is important that you maintain a positive demeanor which will in turn, bring control and calm to the situation. The Proverbs writer tells us that a gentle answer turns away wrath.

—✕✕✕—

It is human tendency to appease the person who is angry.

There are times when you should withdraw from a volatile situation. If you indulge an angry person and keep putting up with this type of behavior, there is a strong possibility that you will become angry. This is a risk that is too big to take and when things become too hot to handle, you must acknowledge that your anger is contrary to what God desires for your life. Right now I can almost visualize the hair on the back of your neck standing straight up. People tell me all the time that their anger is not their own fault but it is the fault of their Latin, Italian, Scottish, Irish, African and Norwegian ancestors. I do not buy that kind of talk. If you want to excuse your anger problem and say you "just can't help it" because your great uncle Theodore gave it to you, you need to stand in front of the mirror, point your finger at yours truly and say out loud to yourself, "Your angry temper does not please God." Then acknowledge that the anger eating you alive is only there because you chose to let it come in and live there.

I am continually amazed when people blame everyone else for their own angry attitude. Guess what. Anger is a learned behavior just like overeating, gambling and drinking. You choose your attitude of anger just as you choose other behaviors. Here is what probably happened that started all of this. One day when you were two years old you got ticked off. You threw your bad self on the floor, kicking, screaming, crying, ranting and raving and you got your way. Then you said, "Wow! This is cool. Every time I want my way, I'll just get mad. I'll huff and puff and tear somebody's head off and scream if I don't like the way things are going." Let me repeat myself. Anger is a learned behavior. It is really quite apparent when you scream like a wild banshee at one of your family members and then you quickly switch on your sweet voice to say, "Hello??" into the ringing telephone. Why don't you just grow up? Why don't you choose a better way? How is it that we can be so cruel and verbally abusive to the people closest to us, yet we would never dream of showing that same nasty face of abuse to others? If our anger was truly genetic we would never have any control. We would be on a wild rampage all the time with no restraints. The truth is that we calculate our anger and we must take responsibility for the anger in our lives. Otherwise, we will never find emotional balance or healing.

We must put a limit on our anger. Again, do not let the sun go down on your wrath. Paul warns us to never let our anger remain. He did not say that we should never feel angry or that we were shallow Christians if we got mad. He simply instructed us to fix our anger before it turns into gangrene and rots our soul. In I Peter 4:8, he tells us to "Keep fervent in love for one another." Love covers a multitude of sins and we must keep our love for Christ alive. If we are passionate about Him, we will love others and be quick to forgive. When we are full of God's grace we can forgive others, even when they have hurt us and are insensitive to the fact that they have done so. Show me someone who has learned to control their anger and I will show you a mature individual. The Proverb tells us that he who is slow to anger has great understanding. When you practice controlling your anger, you show the world that you are growing up. Proverbs 22: 24-25 tells us not to associate with a man given to anger or go with a hot-tempered person lest we learn his ways and snare our souls.

There is an old adage that says you will never know how the other person feels until you walk a mile in their shoes. A root of anger is selfishness. People who think only of themselves and how things affect them are extremely selfish. We should always try to feel what the other person is feeling. It is called empathy. Here is a simple insight. You cannot be empathetic and hostile toward someone at the same time.

You may feel at this point that I have gone overboard on this whole anger section. In fact you are probably saying to yourself at this moment, "I thought this book would help me become healthy, wealthy and wise." To which my reply is, "Well it will! It just takes time to throw out, sort through, organize and then get a fresh start!" My first suggestion is to laugh at yourself. You will get over yourself if you laugh. One of the main characteristics of an angry person is that they take themselves much too seriously. Lighten up. Smile a big, toothless grin. You really need to work on this. You would not care what people thought about you if you knew how seldom they really did. Be good to others and repay evil with good. Romans 12:21 says, "If it's possible, be at peace with all men and never take your own revenge." In other words, learn to take the high road. It is so difficult when people say mean things. We want to say mean things back. Practice the Golden Rule. Matthew 7:12 instructs us to do unto others as we would have them do unto us. Why? What does this have to do with anger issues? Here is the answer: we feel good when we do the right thing and the right thing is to forgive. We must practice forgiveness until we perfect it. We do this by giving up our rights. Ephesians 4:32 says, "Be ye kind to one another, tenderhearted, forgiving one another."

> You would not care what people thought about you if you knew how seldom they really did.

People who are angry have deep-rooted problems in their lives.

At the core of those problems is an unwillingness to forgive. This unforgiving spirit is like fuel on a fire as it feeds on anger and ultimately rages uncontrollably. This is also a choice we must make. We are in the judge's seat. We often assess the situation and/or the offending person and decide that they do not deserve forgiveness. The Apostle Paul appeals to us in his writings to be kind one to another and forgive as God forgives us.

Jesus Christ gave us the pristine example on releasing our rights. He gave up his throne, his status, his life and he forgave us. People who demand and defend their rights are the people who have never surrendered their lives to the lordship of Jesus Christ. These people are control freaks. They are terrified to let go and give up their rights to God or anyone else. They have built up a fortified bunker with cement and steel walls. There are Sherman tanks lined up all the way around their hearts as they scream, "Just try to get close to me and I'll blast you back!" Defensive? Oh, absolutely. These same people wonder why they never grow spiritually. Go figure. It is the very same thing that keeps them from getting over their anger and giving up their rights to God.

So, how DO we resolve our anger problem? In a nutshell, we give up our rights. We ask for forgiveness and we restore our relationships with those who have offended us. There are obviously situations when restoring a relationship would be detrimental and asinine for all involved. For instance, the abused should not attempt to strike up a relationship with their abuser. However, the rest of us need to grow up, deal with it, get over it and move on. When we do this, we break up that fallow ground in our hearts and God re-seeds the soil with fresh grace and power for us to live a Wholly Fit Life.

Since you have likely become quite used to all my little lists and self-evaluation tests in this book, I am going to offer you another. Here are some helpful tidbits on dealing with the "before, during and after" of an angry confrontation.

When angry people confront you, take note of your reaction. Do you immediately empathize with them to your detriment? Do you feel depressed or anxious? Before you rush to placate their feelings or keep the peace, remind yourself that no matter how angry the other person may be, you are NOT required to respond or react! Their anger is *their* problem and ultimately, they must decide what to do with it. It is not about you, Baby! You have already done your part by remaining calm and not reacting.

Be careful not to criticize the other person. Start by expressing how you feel about the situation instead of taking a defensive stance and blaming the other person. This will create a feeling of openness and safety for the other person. Lead by good example and let them know you are listening to what they have to say. Once they realize you are listening, they should reciprocate and respond in a civilized manner.

If you find yourself in the midst of an explosive or hostile conflict with someone, please walk away. Nothing productive will occur when both parties are screaming at each other. Besides, neither party is listening to what the other has to say.

Sit down when you have time to process your emotions. Express your feelings by writing in a journal. It allows you to completely and fully express all of your emotions regarding the situation. It also brings unresolved anger to the surface. The writing part is essential because your paper will listen and your little journal is not going to scream back at you, I promise!

The classic outcome of repressed anger is dangerous because it often leads to depression. I understand that there are those who feel that the hope of Christ in us should resolve every physical, mental and emotional problem we may have and that we should not seek other cures. First and foremost, I believe that we should pray about every situation in our lives. However, after praying, if the symptoms of depression continue, we need to seek wise counsel and not be afraid to take the appropriate medications. Case in point: if I have a kidney infection, I must take antibiotics to rid myself of the poison inside my body. Just as important, if I am depressed, I may need medication to help correct the chemical imbalance in my brain. Depression IS real and is not something you can just turn on or off. Depression can descend on all of us like a black curtain. It can be debilitating and leave us feeling hopeless and despairing. It is saddening when self-righteous people with a Pharisaical attitude begin to bad mouth others who are dealing with depression. We are the people of God and we need to show mercy to those in need rather than grinding them into the ground and mocking them in the midst of our own denial. Please just stop pretending. We are all human! No matter how "high-and-mighty" people think they are as they peer down at the rest of us from their number nine cloud, they really do walk amidst us, as evidenced by the dirty, blackened soles of their feet which dangle from above.

The World Health Organization lists depression as the second leading cause of disability related to illness. There are more than eleven million people who take medication for depression. Depression can be situationally induced and may last for months, weeks, and even years. Some people have dealt with depression their entire lives, yet have never felt the freedom to discuss it because it feels embarrassing and shameful. It also makes people feel isolated and very alone in their depressed state of mind.

Let's leave the clinical aspect of depression and focus on the emotional side. When I say that I feel sad or discouraged, it actually makes me feel sad and discouraged. My eyes lose their brightness. My heart slows and there is an overall feeling of negativity and defeat. We cannot afford to let our feelings control the way we act or think because feelings are unreliable. When we give in to our feelings, we literally create the opportunity to become moody and withdrawn. Generally speaking, we dig the pit and then fall in headfirst. We lose perspective. Once again, let's refer back to Elijah. He was God's superhero. One day he had a big showdown at the top of Mt. Carmel with a bunch of Queen Jezebel's guys. He was radically militant with his approach to showing whose God was the true God. When reading the account of Elijah versus the Bunch of Baal Bullies, I feel electrified by his display of confidence. He ordered fire down from Heaven and fire fell. A few days later, however, his world crumbled when he heard that Jezebel had sent her henchmen bomb squad to do him in. Next we see him deflated, depressed, and diagnosing himself as bipolar and paranoid. He wanted to give up and die and he felt like nobody cared about him in his fight to defend Jehovah God. Imagine that! He had a meltdown just like we have today!

Depression often comes to us during or after life-changing events. Whether the event or circumstance is positive or negative, we experience an emotional letdown. It is in these times that we have a tendency to waiver emotionally. However, it is also essential during this same time that we pray on the whole armor of God. Verse 2 of I Kings 19 is an eye opener. Elijah, the fearless man of God turned into a terrified coward and ran away into the desert. Instead of looking at the full facts and getting a true perspective on the situation, Elijah began to analyze what happened and he withdrew. Elijah made four mistakes. (1) He focused on feelings rather than facts. (2) He compared himself to others. (3) He blamed himself and (4) He exaggerated the negative.

Elijah felt like a loser, a coward and a failure. Sometimes we feel just like Elijah felt and we become depressed when we give in to how we feel instead of looking at the facts. Delusion is a strong, blinding, thick fog that obscures our vision. I was flying into New York recently with both of my eyes tightly shut. The airplane was pitching and bucking so much that I felt like I was getting my neck adjusted and my spine realigned. The real white-knuckle moment came when we began our final approach to solid ground. All I could see when I built up enough courage to open my eyes was white, blinding fog. I had absolutely no concept of where our airplane was in relation to the ground, nor did I know how we were going to get there and I felt terrified.

Elijah did exactly what we do. He judged the situation in his life based on how he felt and by the frame of mind the circumstances put him in. We cannot and should not do this. However, because we are human, it happens to every one of us. Consequently, we must remind ourselves daily that God is still in control.

We do not have to live depressed. We can live an abundant, joyful life. If I have a broken foot, I cannot run, no matter how much I want to do so. I am simply not able. I am incapable of fully functioning and doing everything I normally do. Depression is very much the same. When we become depressed, something is broken inside of our brain. There is often a chemical imbalance which causes a breakdown of communication in the brain. If you are in deep depression, you are probably thinking as you read this, "You don't know. You could not possibly understand what I am dealing with." And my reply to that is this: you are right. I probably have no way of comprehending your pain, but let me bring hope to your situation. I have been close to people who have come through horrific, life-altering tragedies. I have watched in amazed wonder at their heroic responses. A friend of mine who was sexually abused as a little girl for many years by several family members found the courage and strength to forgive her abusers. She has now become one of the most powerful leaders of women in the 21st century. She had a choice to make. She could have decided that her life was wretched, ruined, finished, and that she was a shattered and shamed victim whose innocence had been destroyed. Instead, she allowed her past to shape, mold and make her character into something pristine and beautiful.

I have watched my mother embrace the sorrow and grief over the past several months due to the loss of her beautiful son. In absolute blinding trust, she has turned from her suffering heart to look into the face of God, proclaiming his faithful, steadfast love and holding onto the promise that His grace is sufficient to carry her through. While having a cup of tea with her one day, I admitted to her that the loss of my brother was overwhelming and that I cry often. I then asked her how she was doing and she replied, "Oh, yes, Nan. I cry too." She continued, "Sometimes I wake up in the early morning hours and it's like a black, dense fog of depression tries to roll in and cover me up, but I say out loud, 'no way! This will not control my thoughts!' and then I worship God. I get up and command my feet to walk and my hands to work. I refuse to allow depression to rule my day and my mind. I set my heart on things above. I lift my eyes to the hills from whence cometh my help. I am committed to bless the Lord at all times. I will continually give thanks for his excellent greatness to me and our beautiful family."

> We must remind ourselves daily that God is still in control.

The second mistake Elijah made (which we make too) was comparing himself to others. Elijah said, "It is enough now, Lord. Take my life for I am no better than my father." Elijah felt that his life was in vain and that he did not count for anything. In II Corinthians 10:12, the Apostle Paul said that it is unwise for us to compare ourselves to others. You are unique. God made you with a special design. After you were born, there has never been another duplicate. You broke the mold! You really are one in a million, so stop looking at others and feeling less than important. You are priceless! On the other end of the spectrum are high-and-mighty people who compare themselves to others. They are full of themselves and arrogant. This is unhealthy. They need to chill out and be themselves. Nobody can be anyone except themselves and if anyone tries to be someone else, depression will most likely set in. I have a friend who says, "I tried to be somebody else, but everybody else was taken, so I decided to just be myself." You do not need to be a better someone else. You just need to be a better you.

The third mistake Elijah made was that he blamed himself. When we are depressed, we feel guilty about everything that seems wrong and we think we are the reason. Elijah thought, by obeying God that everything would turn out as he planned. He thought it was a done deal. After the fire fell, just as planned, Israel would return to Jehovah God. Jezebel would turn from her wicked ways and become the Golden Girl who would build new housing developments for the less fortunate. To the dismay of Elijah, none of this transpired. As a matter of fact, Ms. Jezzie went on a witch hunt for the faithful prophet and she sent word that she would kill him within 72 hours.

I wish I could have given Elijah a heads up like I am trying to give you. We cannot take responsibility for other people's bad choices or for their lack of desire to do the right thing. As parents, we must learn this lesson. If we do not, there is a strong possibility of becoming chronically discouraged and clinically depressed. Our children develop their own temperaments, their own wills, and their own distinct personalities. We can influence them, love them, and pour our lives into them. We can do everything possible to help them have a good life. Guess what. They may still make bad decisions, choose the wrong friends and the wrong spouses. They may even walk down the pathway of devastating temptation which sets them up for a downward spiral. You think you can control them? Absolutely not. We will be deeply depressed and unfulfilled as we descend into the pit of washed-up parenthood. Forget it. We have done everything we could to influence them, love them and believe in them. We have given them our very best. Now it is time to let them go. At some point, people must take responsibility for their own actions.

The fourth mistake Elijah made was exaggerating the negative. Feel free to read about Elijah's "Prozac Moment" in I Kings 19:10. Elijah was whining to God and recounting all of his own great feats of steadfast faithfulness. Listen in with me as he vents to God. (We have all been here, so do not get all smug and high-and-mighty). Allow me to paraphrase the King James Version into the Nancy G. version. "I have been true blue to you, Jehovah. Loyal to the bad bone. All of your kids have turned and high-tailed it, totally deserting you! They have forgotten all about your wonderful, benevolent gifts that you have so freely given them. They have forgotten about the times you delivered meals on wheels, brought them clouds of comfort, Caribbean sunsets that lasted far longer than 24 hours and Hawaiian island mega waves, piled up just so they wouldn't get their feet wet. I don't get it! Then they kill off all your good men and here I am on assignment with nobody else standing. It's just me all by myself."

God spoke to the prophet, Elijah, as he speaks to us today. Take a breath. You need to chill out for a little while. When we are at the end of our ropes, we need to rest, relax, eat, and be restored. We will gain a clear perspective on our circumstances only after we are able to pull ourselves back together. It is critical to understand that we are not on our own. God is with us. He is working for our good. Even if we crash and burn and all of the virtue has gone out of our lives, we must remember that God loves us as we are. He comes running to find us wherever we are. He listens and understands because He knows the very motions of our hearts.

It may seem as if I have given you a criss-crossed approach to depression, but I felt that in order to deliver a clear picture, it was important to explore both the symptoms and effects of depression.

FORGIVENESS

It has been building for years - too many years, in fact, to even count.

Consequently, you are now a certified professional at dragging your hurts around and burying them under layers of denial. Do you want to know what my first clue was? Well, let me lay it out for you. You have shopped and shopped and shopped and your credit score is shot to pieces because of excessive debt. You have eaten a truckload of gelato (or perhaps your preference is Häagen-Dazs ice cream). Whatever choice you made, your tummy is now telling on you. You have become reclusive in your relationships and have perhaps even signed up as a closet cyberspace eavesdropper. Why? Because you have been beaten up, bruised and broken to the point that it has left you holding a grudge bigger, deeper and wider than you could ever admit. It kills you a little bit more with each passing day. It is taking your joy, your song, your dance and your laugh. Do you remember when you felt free? When you felt light? When you would break out into a crazy little jig and you didn't give a rip if the whole neighborhood thought you had lost your marbles? What on earth happened to that person you used to be? Unforgiveness happened.

Some serious obstacles which keep us from forgiving and healing are self-pity, anger, fear, pride, revenge, insecurity, holding a grudge and being unwilling to let go of our hurts. There is a reason some people have a beatific glow. Being able to empathize and forgive others can heal your heart and your mind. According to Fred Lufkin, Stanford University Psychologist and author of Forgive for Good, "Holding onto hurt and nursing grudges wears you down physically and emotionally." Forgiving someone can be a powerful antidote.

Charlotte Vanoyen Witvliet, an assistant professor of psychology at Hope College in Holland, Michigan asked 71 volunteers to remember a past hurt. Tests recorded deep spikes in blood pressure, heart rate and muscle tension, the exact responses which occur when people are angry. When the researchers asked those same volunteers to imagine empathizing and even forgiving the people who had wronged them, they were calm by comparison.

According to Lufkin, director of the Stanford Forgiveness Project, forgiveness can be learned. "We teach people to re-write their stories in their minds. To change from being the victim to the hero. If the hurt is from a spouse's unfaithfulness, we often encourage them to think of themselves, not only as a person who was wronged, but as the person who fought to keep the marriage together."

—𝓂𝓋—

Being able to empathize and forgive others can heal your heart and your mind.

Lufkin put his method to the test on five women whose sons had been murdered. After one week of forgiveness training, the women's sense of hurt measured by psychological tests had fallen by more than half. They found they were also less likely to feel depressed and angry. "Forgiving is not about condoning what happened," said Lufkin, "it is about breaking free of the person who wronged us." The sooner we forgive, the better we are.

A survey of 1,423 adults by the University of Michigan for Social Research found that people who had forgiven someone in their past also reported being in better health than those who did not. While 75% felt sure that God had forgiven them for their past mistakes, only 52% had been able to find it in their hearts to forgive others. Alexander Pope very succinctly told us, "to err is human, to forgive divine." In other words, when people do things the wrong way, we need to forgive them because everyone makes mistakes.

The ancient Chinese philosopher, Confucius, said, "Those who cannot forgive others break the bridge over which they themselves must pass." And Nancy Grandquist says, "Forgiveness is the healing balm for broken hearts and broken relationships." If you want to know forgiveness in your life, then you must learn to first forgive.

Almost all emotional pain (along with that famous buzz word, "stress,") comes from unresolved conflict. If we are transparent enough to look at the bare bone facts, we will recognize that it is our willfulness and our stubborn, prideful attitudes that keep us from the resplendent posture of humility and the unfeigned blessing of charitable kindness and longsuffering. Ernest Hemingway wrote a short story called The Capital of the World which takes place in Spain and illustrates my point perfectly. The father and son had been estranged for many years and the father wanted his son to know that he loved him and wished for their relationship to be healed. His son's name was Paco. The father put an ad in the Madrid paper and it read, "Dear Paco, meet me in front of the newsstand tomorrow at noon. All is forgiven." The next day at noon, there were over 800 boys gathered in front of the news agency. I am afraid there are a lot of Pacos in our families, churches, communities and in the world. A mark of greatness is to forgive and keep forgiving, for true forgiveness is a perpetual process (that was another cool quote by me!!). I am reminded of an Irish poem, "May those who love us, love us and those who don't love us, may God turn their hearts. And if he doesn't turn their hearts, may he turn their ankles so we will know them by their limping."

People who find it hard to forgive do not see themselves realistically. They do not see their humanity. They have forgotten that they are merely mortal, after all. They pretend that they have never sinned, failed, or made a mistake. People who refuse to forgive ultimately hurt themselves more than they hurt others. We are not made to sustain and hold onto long term hurts or grudges. When Richard Nixon took a seat next to the widow of Hubert Humphrey at his funeral, people were stunned. This was at Hubert Humphrey's own request and it was shocking because of all the things that had transpired between these two powerful men during the huge political disgrace of Watergate. Three days before Hubert Humphrey died, a close friend walked into his hospital room. He heard Hubert Humphrey talking on the phone and this is what he overheard. "From this vantage point, with the sun setting in my life, all the political speeches, crowds, conventions and the great fights are behind me now. At a time like this, you are forced to deal with your irremediable essence. You are forced to grovel with that which is really important to you. What I have concluded about life is this: when all is said and done, we must forgive each other, redeem each other and move on."

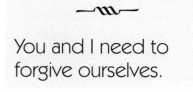

You and I need to forgive ourselves.

The word, "redeem" in the Merriam Webster Dictionary is worth its weight in gold. Redeem means to ransom, free, or rescue. And this is the very best part. It means to remove the obligation of payment or to convert into something of great value. That is exactly what we do when we forgive and forgive and forgive and then forgive again. We redeem the situation, the person, and the one who brought the hurt. This same principle applies to us personally. You and I need to forgive ourselves. We need to understand that Christ brought full redemption. He died and gave His life so that we would revel in the beautiful state of grace. He forgave us and he continues to forgive us in order to redeem us. We are free as a giddy, barefoot child running through fields of green clover in early spring. Live free! Forgive freely.

A dear friend of mine, Kaye Singleton, who to me has proven to be the embodiment of love, grace, and forgiveness, sent me these words. "In the middle of forgiveness is 'give.' Forgiveness is a gift when given to those who have brought us harm. Give the perfect gift every time. Give forgiveness." Here are five steps to help us forgive.

1.   Remember all the forgiveness you have received from God. If we acknowledge what God has done for us, we will not have a problem forgiving others.

2. Realize that forgiveness is a choice, not an emotion. We must take the first step and emotion most often will follow.

3. Understand the consequences of not forgiving the offender. Until we forgive the person that hurt us, they will continue to have power over us. We will be ill emotionally, physically, and spiritually. Letting go of our hurtful past will revitalize our future.

4. Forgive the person right now. We must not allow another moment to pass as we may never have another opportunity.

5. Look at the problem as a potential for growth. Hurts and devastation can be the stepping stones that lead to great strength and wisdom.

Make forgiveness happen by putting down the old script and writing something new. Let your response be something entirely different than ever before. If you see a blowout coming, try first to analyze the situation and ask yourself these questions. Does this really matter? What is this really all about? Can I do things differently? Remember, you have choices that you can make and you can decide how you will respond. I cannot change the circumstances. I cannot even change the other person, but I can control and change the way I react. When I change, the situation will change. I hold the power. I can choose to change and be empowered to grow through the process of forgiving.

PEACE

Colossians 3:15 tells us to let the peace of God rule our hearts. We need to grab hold of this scripture and actually *allow* the peace of God to rule our hearts. When we abide in Him and our hearts are filled with His presence, we will know peace. I was startled to find that the word "rule" literally means "umpire." I enjoy going to my grandboys' games. I am completely interested in whatever sport they are playing, soccer, basketball, or baseball. It's all fun to me. Besides, I love the popcorn and the Hot Tamales from the snack shack. I am always relieved that I am not in charge of making the calls in a game, especially when there is a play that is unclear and no one knows exactly what took place. I would be a biased umpire if the runner was my grandson, Taylor, who slid into home base to meet the catcher who was already there holding the ball with his foot on the base. I would be up in the stands screaming, "It was a tie! I saw it! It *was* a tie and the tie goes to the runner!" This is the way I would call it, albeit incorrect. One thing I am sure of and grateful for is that God is fair. He always does the right thing and He always makes the right call. He is sovereign and we can trust in the knowledge that He will do what is best for our lives. Let Him make the call.

It is impossible for us to have peace in the network of our lives until we have absolute peace on the inside. We all experience times in our lives when we are troubled by a decision we must make, but we must not allow ourselves to procrastinate. Indecisiveness brings confusion which multiplies frustration and breeds fear, anxiety, and panic attacks. James 1:8 says, "A double-minded man is unstable in all his ways." In the New Living Translation, James 1:5 tells us that if we need wisdom and we want to know what God wants us to do, just ask Him. He will gladly tell us. He will not resent our asking. We must be sure, though, that we really expect an answer and we must be ready to accept whatever that answer might be. A double-minded man or woman is as unsettled as the wave of the sea that is driven and tossed by the wind. Unsettled people, then, should not expect to receive anything from the Lord. They cannot make up their minds. They waver back and forth in everything they do. We reach decisions by prayerful consideration and seeking God and we then need to commit to those decisions.

Let your final decision truly count. Make up your mind. Be decisive and strong. Don't do any of that "tossed by the wind, driven by the ocean waves" stuff. You could really get seasick, you know. If you are desperate to find peace, do not prolong your decision. Yes, you should pause, focus your heart, and listen. In doing so, God will bring you the answer. I have met the most miserable, irritable, unhappy people and the basis of their negative attitude is indecisiveness. They cannot decide which side they want to part their hair on and what color it should be this week. They are troubled with whether they should eat peanut butter on their toast, or eat their toast with peanut butter. Their lives are totally and completely chaotic. Here is the key: be obedient to God's Word. Live by it. Trust God with the ultimate decisions in your life. When He declares his decision in your circumstance, live by it. No one loves you or cares about you more than He does. Trust Him. He wants you to win. He is the fairest umpire I know. Let Him rule your life and then give yourself the gift of perfect peace.

Before I close this chapter on emotional wellness, I feel compelled to leave you with a few words about being thankful. We have so much to be grateful for. A heart full of thanks and gratitude is one that emits the sweetest of fragrances. We all face disappointments and heartbreak. We fail God and others and often we fail ourselves. It is good and right that we live with sincere humility just in case we need a coup de' grace, which is a stroke of mercy. We should always be quick to pour out our love and mercy on those who are hurting and have lost their way. How can they find their way back if we do not leave a trail of tears, compassion and gentle mercy?

I have made several trips to South Africa and have discovered through personal experience that the Africans are beautiful people. I came across this wonderful story and I want to share it with you. In Southern Africa there is a tribe called Babemba. In this tribe, if it is discovered that a person has done something wrong which could destroy their delicate social bond, all work in the village comes to an immediate halt. The people in the tribe gather around the offender and one by one, begin to recite everything he or she has done right in their life, including every good deed, thoughtful behavior, and every act of social responsibility. Everything spoken about the person must be true and spoken honestly. The time honored consequence of misbehavior is to appreciate that person back into the better part of themselves. The offending person is given a chance (coup de' grace) to remember who they really are and why they are valuable and important to the life of the village. What kind of world would we know if we practiced and perpetuated this kind of thinking? It is up to us to model the attitude of benevolent gratitude, love and thankfulness. It will change us and our world, one life at a time. Someone shared with me recently that your level of gratitude is in direct proportion to the amount of forgiveness and healing that has come into your life. A lot of sin followed by a lot of healing equals a lot of gratitude, which again, emits the sweetest of fragrances.

9

beautifully Natural

Hair, Skin and Nails

HAIR

You may be sick of me telling you this, but I must be forthright. It is all about nutrition. It is all about less sugar and less flour. Now, are you ready for this? A lack of nutrition in addition to an onslaught of sugary desserts, drinks, and white flour brings on a lot of scary symptoms. By the time I had delivered my fourth child, I thought I was going to have to purchase a wig for my Easter hair-do. During my pregnancies, my hair grew and was thick and healthy. A few months after the babies were born, however, my hair fell out in clumps. I was relieved to learn that this is a normal process due to a hormone that inhibits hair loss during pregnancy. A deficiency of Vitamin A may also cause hair to be dull, dry and lusterless. Eventually, it may begin to fall out. A deficiency of manganese may slow the growth of hair. Hair is composed mostly of protein. A deficiency of protein in the diet can result in a temporary change of hair color and texture. Now, this is pretty amazing. Do you know you can sometimes have a return of your normal hair color even after your hair has turned grey? This may happen by taking appropriate amounts of copper, folic acid, pantothenic acid, and/or paraominobenzoil acid (PABA). Five mgs

of folic acid and 300 mgs of PABA and pantothenic acid along with
B complex vitamins have been shown to prevent hair loss and to
restore hair color.

Wonderful, beautiful hair needs several contributions. If at all
possible, try to have a scalp massage every week. Better yet, have
your best friend brush your hair (it's less expensive!). Brush it until
it shines and you feel your scalp sit up and say, "WOW!" Always use
a wide tooth comb on just-shampooed locks. No brushing. This is
a hair felony or at least a misdemeanor. It breaks your hair off and
causes major split ends. Also, there is a huge difference between
those cheap $.97 products and the more expensive ones. If you can
afford to buy the more expensive hair products, please do so because
your hair is worth the extra money. The more expensive products
often go on sale, so watch for the good deals at Marshalls or TJ
Maxx. There are also many great leave-in treatments that mend and
soothe dry, split ends. Try not to use hot rollers or hair dryers on
your hair every day. Let it rest. Even God took a day off. Your hair
should have one too.

SKIN

Beauty IS more than skin deep. Your skin says a lot about what is
going on inside of you. The stuff you eat. The stuff you think. The
stuff you speak. It is all showing on your skin. So, here is a daily
remedy for happy skin. Water. Hydrate. Water. Hydrate. Breathe,
breathe, breathe. Eat fresh veggies, fresh fruit, nuts and berries and
fast once a week. I recommend a three day fast every eight to ten
weeks. Fasting is not just for your spiritual well being. It benefits our
physical bodies in a huge way. Do you want your skin to glow? I am
not talking about that brown bronzer stuff that leaves orange stripes
under your chin and a crease beside your ears that makes you look like
a leftover jack-o-lantern. If you really want skin that looks alive and
transparent, here it is in a nutshell. Exercise. Get enough sleep. Rest

seven to eight hours a night. Drink half of the Hoover Dam reserve. Fast often. Breathe deep, cleansing, refreshing breaths. Think pure, right thoughts. You will have the Mary Kay representative asking for your autograph and your skin secrets. I have tried most every line of cosmetic creams and lotions that are on the market. Many of the products advertised in magazines and sold in department stores are marketed mostly by their impressive packaging. While there is a difference in cheap versus expensive hair products, it is my humble opinion that this is not necessarily the case with skin products. I am convinced that you can get the same results from Brand X at Walgreens that you get from that $700 jar of the promised "miracle cream." The secret is truly taking care of your skin *every* day.

Many of our skin's stories are told by the lives we live and the people we are related to. The mothers of my sons-in-law both come from a long line of American Native Indian tribes. They have perfectly beautiful, wrinkle-free faces and maybe one or two hairs in their heads that are threatening to turn two shades lighter than dark. It is all in the genetics, no matter whether you are thick-skinned, thin-skinned, or whether you have dry or oily skin. Our skin is also affected by the elements we are exposed to. I believe in serious sun damage control. I put on moisturizer with 58 SPF every morning and if I am going to be in the sun, I always wear a hat. I am religious about this. I have had a few trips to the skin cancer doctor, all related to my young, sun-tanned baby oiled, bake-your-brains-out days. Please do NOT take your gorgeous skin down to the tanning beds and broil yourself like a red lobster. Chances are that in ten or fifteen years you will be forced to buy yourself a new nose. Why would you want to do that when you look so great in the one you have now?

Here are six recipes for yummy aromatherapy baths that will make our skin happy:

Skin-Smoothing Citrus Bath

—ɯɯ—

Ingredients: 1 navel orange; 1 cup of whole, divided cloves; 1 cup pulp-free orange juice; ½ cup soy milk; and 2 teaspoons lavender essential oil.

How to make it: Cut orange into even slices; insert ½ cup cloves into slices. Fill tub with hot water; add oranges, remaining ½ cup cloves, orange juice, soy milk, and lavender oil.

Why it's good for you: It is rich in antioxidants and vitamins A and C. Citrus-fruit acids are natural exfoliants and soften skin while preventing free radical damage. While soaking, use a washcloth to slough off dead skin cells loosened by the fruit acids. Cloves enhance the sensory experience.

Best time to soak: Anytime you need a lift. Citrus scents have been shown to make people feel happier, and the lavender abates stress.

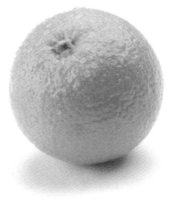

Hydrating Milk Bath for Sensitive Skin

Ingredients: 1 cup dry milk; ½ cup cornstarch; ¼ cup dried lavender sprigs.

How to make it: Combine dry milk and cornstarch in a bowl; pour mixture into hot, running water. Once tub is full, scatter lavender sprigs in water.

Why it's good for you: Milk contains lactic acid, a natural exfoliant that softens skin by dissolving rough patches. It is also loaded with moisturizing proteins and vitamins. The cornstarch gives the bath water a silky feeling.

Best time to soak: When your skin is dull and flaky, or right before bed to encourage a pleasant night's sleep.

Beware: Milk can leave the tub slippery, so be sure to rinse the residue after finishing your bath.

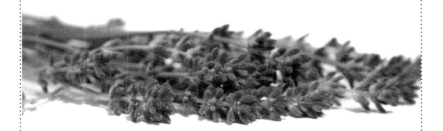

Creativity-Boosting Bath

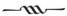

Ingredients: 2 capfuls of Colour Energy Liquid Colour Bath in Violet (fragrance-free mix of organic pigments, glycerin, and water; available at www.ColourEnergy.com.

How to make it: Add liquid to hot water; surround tub with violet candles and flowers to bolster effects. Concentrate on color while soaking.

Why it's good for you: The perks of this bath are more emotional than physical. Color affects your mood, energy level, and overall sense of well-being and violet is said to inspire creativity.

Best time to soak: When you are in a creative rut or need to make a big decision.

Beware: If used alone, it will not stain your tub. If mixed with other bath products, it may. If this happens, clean your tub with baking soda and water.

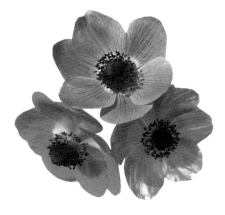

Nourishing Marine Bath for the Chronic Cold Catcher

Ingredients: ½ cup **Nutrex Hawaiian Spirulina Pacifica Powder** (available at grocery and health-food stores); 6 drops of citrus essential oils, such as bergamot and lime; 12 small orchids.

How to make it: Pour spirulina powder mixture into hot water. Next, add oils and float your flowers.

Why it's good for you: Spirulina is a blue-green algae that is rich in proteins, antioxidants, vitamins, and essential fatty acids. When absorbed, it stimulates circulation and metabolism, flushing fluids from cells and replacing them with minerals to deliver soft, glowing skin. It also fights fatigue and bolsters the immune system.

Best time to soak: When you feel sluggish or sick.

Beware: If you have shellfish allergies or a thyroid condition, the iodine in spirulina can irritate skin and alter your thyroid level.

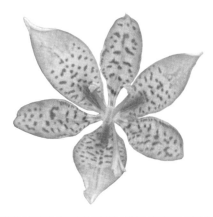

Muscle-Melting Herbal Bath for the Exercise Enthusiast

Ingredients: 1/8 cup crushed basil plus whole basil leaves; 1/8 crushed bay laurel, plus whole laurel leaves for the tub; ¼ cup crushed rosemary, plus whole sprigs for tub; 1 ounce of jojoba oil.

How to make it: Combine crushed herbs in a muslin pouch or cheesecloth and tie off the top. Place the pouch into the tub while it fills with warm water (not as hot on this bath in order to invigorate the tired muscles); add jojoba oil and whole herbal leaves for an aesthetically pleasing bonus.

Why it's good for you: A combination of cool water and warming herbs awakens the senses and alleviates aches. Rosemary is a well-known analgesic. Bay laurel has proven antiseptic and antibacterial properties.

Best time to soak: After an invigorating exercise or when you feel sore.

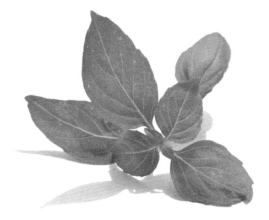

Rejuvenating Rose Bath for Softening the Skin

—⁓—

Ingredients: 3 drops rose essential oil; 1 tablespoon sweet almond oil; ¼ cup rose water; 2 tablespoons organic apple cider vinegar; 1 handful of rose petals.

How to make it: Drizzle rose and almond oils into hot water. Add rose water and apple cider vinegar; gently drop in rose petals.

Why it's good for you: Rose has astringent and is an anti-inflammatory which tones and softens the skin. Sweet almond oil has fatty acids which help the skin maintain moisture and apple cider vinegar neutralizes the pH of the water, ensuring that the essential oils will not cause skin irritation.

Best time to soak: Anytime you want to soften your skin.

Beware: Skip the almond oil if you have a nut allergy.

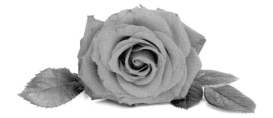

FINGERNAILS

You and I both want strong, healthy fingernails. In fact, it is on my list of things I want when I get to Heaven. I would really like to try out a set of real fingernails that are non-chipped, non-split, and non-refundable…Okay, I may not care once we all get there, but for now I can hope. Okay, let's talk about fake nails. They are totally out. They are a thing of the past just like the ringer washing machine. First and foremost, acrylic, silk and any type of nail wrap kills your nail beds. Here is a visual for you. It would be like wrapping your whole body in five layers of saran wrap, hot-gluing the entire surface and then taking a jack hammer to polish you off. Your nails want to breathe, so let them! Instead, soak your nails for fifteen minutes (once or twice a week) in a nice, fragrant aromatherapy mixture. I use six drops of lavender, six drops of bay, six drops of almond, six drops of grape seed, and six ounces of warm sesame or soy oil. Viola!! Your nails will be happy and they will thank you for keeping them out of the torture tank.

10

Fasting

"The road to health is the one that begins with an understanding and commitment to cleanse and detoxify the body. To restore balance, peace and harmony."

Dr. Bernard Jensen B.C., Ph.D.

Let's talk about fasting for a minute. Just writing that last sentence immediately made my stomach rumble loudly and go into a panic. Regardless of what your Aunt Nellie told you, you will not pass away if you go without food for a day or two and I merely want to point out some very valuable rewards that come with saying "NO" to your belly. Hold it! Here is another disclaimer! If you have any sort of health concerns, right down to the hangnail on your baby toe, please consult your physician before changing your eating habits or participating in a new diet. There are so many wonderful fasts that can kick-start and revitalize our bodies and minds, but we must make sure that both the fast and the timing of the fast are appropriate for our bodies.

If I told you that our bodies are mobile storage bins filled to the brim with cesspools of putrid matter and toxic waste which are all being slowly distributed into our colons, livers and intestines, would

you then feel motivated to do a
cleansing fast?

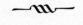

I was completely dumbfounded
when I discovered that there are
over 80,000 chemicals licensed
for commercial use and 2,000
new chemicals are added every
year. No wonder we are in a
constant battle to defend our

Without a doubt,
there are certain
levels of these toxins
that we ingest every
day.

immune systems from these perpetrators. Without a doubt, there
are certain levels of these toxins that we ingest every day. Despite
our best efforts at weight loss, we are being completely sabotaged
by an overstressed toxic liver that is totally bogged down and unable
to appropriately filter the waste. Ultimately, our metabolism comes
to a screeching halt. Alexandra Rome, in her March, 2004 article
published in the San Francisco Chronicle wrote, "We are all in
this chemical soup together. Chemicals in our environment don't
discriminate."

You may look in the mirror and wonder why your face looks sallow,
lifeless and exhausted. One thing is for sure. Your body does not lie.
Here are some clear cut symptoms indicative of massive amounts of
built-up sludge in your system. I want to give you a heads up about
what is going on inside of you. Who knows? Maybe this is the wake-
up call you need to get your burdened body on the path to a vibrant,
healthy you. Do you have acne blemishes, hives or itchy rashes?
Discoloration in the eyes? Red, swollen or teary eyes? Hemorrhoids
or varicose veins? Hormonal imbalances such as PMS, menstrual
problems or hot flashes (power surges)? Heat in your face or eyes?
Gas, bloating, belching, nausea and mild frontal headaches (especially
after eating fatty foods)? Difficulty digesting fats? Loss of appetite
or an eating disorder? Weight gain even when you are controlling
your food intake? Tiredness or sleepy after eating? Tendency to wake

up between 1:00 and 3:00 a.m.? Weak tendons, ligaments or muscles? Pain under the right shoulder blade? Excessive, unexplained or sudden bursts of anger, irritability or rage? Depression disproportionate to life events? Elevated liver enzymes (SGOT, SGPT)? High bilirubin levels? Whether you have one or all of these symptoms, your body is sending you a big SOS. You need to consider a fast, whether it is water or juice. Do you have bad breath or body odor? A frequent, bitter taste in your mouth? A coated tongue? Putrid and/or painful gas? Problems with elimination? Constipation or diarrhea? Long, thin, or foul-smelling stool with undigested food particles? Lower back pain? Abdominal discomfort or fullness? Rectal itching? Bruises that do not heal? Difficulty perspiring? Joint aches or pains? Arthritis? Colitis or diverticulitis? Systemic yeast infections or problems with Candida? Parasites or worms? Multiple allergic response syndrome (MARS)? Multiple food allergies or sensitivities to the environment? Sensitivity to perfumes, other fragrances, car fumes or other odors? You need to help your burdened body. You need to flush out and rid your system of all these bombastic toxins.

In addition to all of the preceding symptoms, the following list is a surefire indication that you need a super detox day in your life: frequent cough, stuffy nose, sinus problems, tendency for cold and flu, exhaustion, lethargy and fatigue, mental dullness, poor memory and premature aging.

Now, if you have gone through this extensive list and put a check by a few or even many of these symptoms, chances are that you are feeling overwhelmed and maybe even fearful by now. Please do not despair. This is a good turning point and a good place to start over. You can start right away, so get ready. Prepare to reduce your body's chemical burdens. Let's get straight to the point. Do not call your mother and ask her permission. Just decide that this is your moment and you are turning your life around. This is not about blame, condemnation or guilt. If you are sick or overweight and if you do not have proper energy levels, please be patient as you learn to understand the enemy. There are several battlefronts we should be aware of. We know that our environment is full of toxic, hazardous materials. Let me identify a few of these very common, everyday toxins. The very air we breathe is filthy with pollution and chemicals from industrial companies, automobiles, cigarette smoke, and many other toxins.

The Environmental Protection Agency has documented that there are more than 55,000 chemical dump holes currently in existence in the United States. These are a definite source for potential leakage into our ground water. Our food is loaded with chemical fertilizers and additives and is contaminated by lead and aluminum cans and containers. D. Lindsey Berkson, a bioenvironmentalist educated at Tulane University, reveals a shocking associated press story in her book, *Hormone Deception*. It seems that toxic, heavy metals such as cadmium, lead and arsenic along with dioxins and perhaps even radioactive wastes are routinely used to fertilize our fields. For example, in Gore, Oklahoma (I would not want to live in that city), there is a low level of radioactive waste that is prevalent from a nearby uranium processing plant. This plant is licensed to produce and sell commercial fertilizer. This same processing plant has sprayed over 9,000 acres of grazing land. Follow my thought here. This land is where our cows munch the new, freshly fertilized grass. We then drink their milk and eat their butter on our toast. No wonder we are a sick nation. The United States does not regulate the use of fertilizers which means that the medical, municipal and industrial waste can be spread over the ground where our crops grow and our cattle graze. You think that's bad? Read this next part. Municipal sewage systems alone, says Berkston, sell some 36% of their 11.6 billion pounds of waste materials to farmers looking for fertilizer.

I have friends who work for a large corporation who recently told me that their job is to melt down chopped pieces of silicone, which, in its liquid form, becomes a toxic acid. This liquid, toxic acid is then converted to a medical grade acid which is then added to our food and drinks as various forms of preservatives. One day, my friend was carrying a large container of this toxic acid. Somehow the container developed a leak. A small drop fell on the top of his boot. In a split second, it melted through the boot and was eating through his foot to his bone. This story is so scary! We wonder why we have cancer and we wonder

You need to love your liver and care about your colon.

why so many people we love are so sick. It is because this same acid that ate through his boot is also being consumed by unsuspecting people on a daily basis. The idea that these corporations are making mega dollars using toxic acids and turning them into something they call "medical grade" is rather terrifying! I really am not trying to freak you out (well maybe just a little). So what is the solution? Detox. FAST. Be committed. Get disciplined. You need to love your liver and care about your colon.

Below is a list of several "love your liver" foods. Even though you may be wrinkling your nose in disgust at the thought of how these will taste, I promise that your liver will thank you after you eat these foods. For the drama queens who cannot bear to taste the foods listed below, please check out the artichoke soup recipe at the back of the book. It is great for your liver and you will absolutely love the taste.

      One small artichoke
      ½ cup cooked asparagus
      ½ cooked or 1 cup raw beets
      2 medium stalks of celery
      1 to 2 cups of dandelion root tea

1 to 2 scoops of whey
1 to 2 tsp of nutritional yeast flakes

Here is a care list for your colon:

1 to 2 tsp. of Psyllium husk in 8 oz. of water
2 to 3 milled or brown flax seed
1 small raw carrot
1 small apple with skin
1 small pear with skin
1 cup of berries

If you are heading into a one-day fast or detoxification, here is an excellent recipe for a Wholly Fit Cocktail. Please remember to stay in close proximity to your bathroom throughout the day!

First, prepare 2 quarts of cranberry water by adding 8 oz. of unsweetened cranberry juice to 56 oz. of filtered water or add 3 tbsp unsweetened cranberry juice concentrate to 60 oz. of filtered water. Recommended brands of unsweetened cranberry juice are Lakewood 100% Organic, Mountain Sun and Knudsen. Recommended brands of unsweetened cranberry juice concentrate are Knudsen and Tree of Life. Be sure to use juice that has no sugar, corn syrup, or other juices added, including apple or grape. Once the cranberry water is ready, set it aside and gather the following ingredients.

½ tsp. of ground cinnamon
¼ tsp. ground nutmeg
½ tsp. ground ginger
¾ cup freshly squeezed orange juice
¼ cup freshly squeezed lemon juice (add at least 1 tsp. Stevia or Lakanto to sweeten)

Next, bring the cranberry water to a light boil and reduce the heat to low. Combine cinnamon, ginger, and nutmeg and put them into a teaball. Add this mixture to the cranberry water. Simmer 15 to 20 minutes and then cool to room temperature. Stir in the orange and lemon juices. Add Stevia or Lakanto at this time, if desired.

Alternate drinking one cup (8 oz.) of filtered water to 1 ½ cups (12 oz.) of Wholly Fit Cocktail during the day. Drink at least 72 oz. of filtered water throughout the day in addition to the Wholly Fit Cocktail. Make sure you drink at least one cup of liquid every hour. When your feet hit the floor running, here is the schedule.

> Start at 6 a.m. with one cup of filtered water.
> 7 a.m.: 1 cup of Wholly Fit Cocktail.
> 8 a.m.: 1 cup of filtered water.
> 9 a.m.: 1 cup of Wholly Fit Cocktail.
> 10 a.m.: 1 cup of filtered water.
> 11 a.m.: 1 cup of Wholly Fit Cocktail.
> 12 p.m.: 1 cup of filtered water.
> 1 p.m.: 2 cups of Wholly Fit Cocktail.
> 2 p.m.: 1 cup of filtered water.
> 3 p.m.: 1 cup of Wholly Fit Cocktail.
> 4 p.m.: 1 cup of filtered water.
> 5 p.m.: 1½ cups of Wholly Fit Cocktail.
> 6 p.m.: 1 cup of filtered water;
> 7 p.m.: 1 cup of Wholly Fit Cocktail.
> 8 p.m.: 1 cup of filtered water
> 9 p.m.: 1 cup of Wholly Fit Cocktail
> 10 p.m.: 1 cup of filtered water.

Now, let's talk about how to cope with hunger. You may feel hunger pangs when you fast or you may hear a roar erupt from the pit of your stomach. Try not to focus on the feeling of emptiness. Understand that we will often feel an emotional desire as opposed to actually being hungry. I find the first few days of a fast are usually the most challenging. It may seem difficult, but there are so many wonderful benefits that come with a cleansing fast. Do not be discouraged in moments of hunger or weakness, but strengthen your resolve by focusing on all of the positive benefits that will come from the fast. Instead, think about the redemption of your tired intestinal tract as it receives fresh nutrients and is purified and reinstated back to its finest working order.

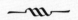

Take a walk. Write in your journal. Read scriptures and pray.

As you deny yourself food, try to do the same with all electronic media. Unplug from the mad rush of your life. Take a walk. Write in your journal. Read scriptures and pray. Get a pedicure or a massage (this will expedite the process of breaking down and ridding your system of toxins). Soak in a tub of organic salts or oils. Listen to soft, beautiful praise music. Worship your creator. Hear the music inside of your heart. Fill your mind with soothing, calm thoughts. Meditate on God's word. Listen for His voice. You will have clarity in your thought processes. One of the most amazing benefits of a fast is how little sleep you need. As I progress in the fast, I require less sleep. In fact, I find that I am well-rested after only four hours of sleep. My family loves it because I wake up super early and am usually baking homemade yeast rolls or cooking up some delectable dish for them to eat when they finally wake up. I am totally and completely energized, so I organize the entire house, every drawer, cabinet, bookcase, etc. This is because my system is not working so hard to digest and rid itself of waste.

Many times I feel alone when I am on a fast. This is a good thing, for during these alone times, we are able to be introspective. It also allows for a deeper connection between God's Spirit and our spirits as we are cleansed both body and soul.

There are many variations of fasting. You must choose the one that you feel works for you. It is essential that you prepare for a fast by eating lots of fruits and vegetables and drinking ample amounts of water. I highly recommend a 3 to 7 day preparation time. Before embarking on a cleansing regiment, please consult with your physician in order to ensure that you are physically able to do the fast.

I know of several over-the-top, fabulous resort spas and retreats that offer seven to fourteen days of fasting, detoxification, and purification regiments. However, since I have never had the express pleasure or the money to retreat at such a spa, I have set up my own personal resort at home. Now, I will admit it is tough with the phone ringing, grandkids running in and out of the house, and chickens, dogs, and cats all needing a piece of me, but I give it a real GO. Why don't you? Here's what you need: silence, solitude, quiet time and light, fragrant-smelling candles. Use soft, white towels and a soft, white robe (okay, mine used to be white, but I washed a load of white towels with my green and red Christmas apron which turned everything pink). Invest in pure, organic bath oils. Be careful getting in and out of the tub so that you do not slip and fall. I also suggest using Epsom salt in the water for a relaxing bath and sea salt for scrubbing.

One of my personal regiments during a fast is to take a Dr. Singha's Hot Mustard Bath (you can order this product online at www.drsingha.com) followed by a homemade, holistic body wrap which will allow you to sweat out your impurities. It is totally amazing. First, turn down your bedcovers, lay a towel down and then lay a sheet on top of the towel. Next, before stepping into your tub of water, brush your skin in circular motions toward your heart using a loofah sponge and gentle strokes. When preparing your Dr. Singha bath, use the hottest water your body can stand, but not so hot that you faint when getting up out of the tub. If you try to sue me for fainting, please remember my disclaimer here. I warned you! Soak for at least 15 to 30 minutes. While in the bath, drink as much pure water as possible with fresh lime or lemon slices. Use a beautiful crystal or silver goblet if you have one. I am not a Diva, but this whole experience makes me feel royal and I promise that you will too! When you step out of the tub, wrap yourself in an extra-large towel, then lay on top of your prepared bed. Next, pile on the covers you previously turned down and let the sweat begin! Let it pour! After you have cooled down, go get in the shower and anoint your skin with some type of pure oil or lotion. I highly recommend pure almond or grapeseed aromatherapy oils. I often mix both of these together with a Vitamin E cream. This is very healing and restoring for your whole body and especially great for your skin.

Fasting and skin care go waaaaaaaaaaaaay back. Remember the beauty queen, Esther? She took a year-long bath. Wow. I can hardly get 30 minutes of bath time before someone is knocking on the door saying, "How long are you staying in there??"

People ask me all the time about fasting. There are many variations of fasting. First and foremost, I fast to draw near to God. I discipline my mind and flesh and demand that it refrains from the comfort, fellowship and pleasure that food brings. There is the pure fast which is water only. Unless you are determined to sign up for dialysis, never, never, never try to fast without drinking water. It is better to drink still (not sparkling) water. Another type of fast is the juice fast. This fast includes drinking pure vegetable or fruit juice in addition to water. One of my favorite health fasts is called The Master Cleanser. I add two tablespoons of organic lemon juice, two tablespoons of pure, grade B maple syrup, and a pinch of cayenne pepper to an 8-ounce glass of pure, distilled water. You can drink this cold or hot. Also, for those of you who desire a massive laxative experience (a MAJOR cleanout!) it is recommended that you drink a quart of water with two teaspoons of sea salt. Boil the water and sea salt and then let it cool before drinking. Although there are critics who have not spoken favorably about this fast, I have had excellent results. However, I have **never** done this cleanse for more than 14 days, nor do I advise it without a doctor's recommendation. There are many other types of fasts available for your physical health. A few are the lymphatic cleanse, the liver cleanse, and the colon cleanse. Again, I suggest that you consult your doctor before beginning any type of health fast.

Before my sweet brother, David, who so courageously battled cancer, passed away, he consulted with Dr. Robert Morse, N.D., D.Sc., I.D., M.H., the creator and founder of God's Herbs Botanical Company in Port Charlotte, Florida. Dr. Morse recommended a 50-day grape juice fast for David. As it turned out, though, my brother did not even have 50 days left to live and we were very disheartened to learn that his cancer was too far advanced to benefit from Dr. Morse's highly acclaimed, therapeutic and healing grape juice regiment. If you or someone you love has been diagnosed with cancer, or any other debilitating disease, I strongly encourage you

Consult your doctor before beginning any type of health fast.

to consider this fast and contact Dr. Morse for a consultation. The recipe for the fast is below and a juicer is necessary for this fast.

This recipe is very simple. Juice one quart of grapes, including the seeds and small stems. Any type of grape is ok, but dark seeded grapes are the best. Try to use organic grapes. They are high in anti-oxidants and have astringent properties. A five to ten day grape juice fast is beneficial. Grapes and lemons are the greatest lymphatic cleansers and cancer busters. Combine this fast with a raw food diet and drink as much grape juice as you want, but again, I highly recommend you contact Dr. Morse.

Cleansing and detoxification are two of the most basic principles for having a healthy body, living longer, fuller lives, looking and feeling fabulous and staying disease-free. If you are faithful to fasting and body cleansing, you will have a better chance of preventing sickness and disease which come as the years accumulate.

11

foods to Put in

Your Wholly Fit Grocery Cart

HERE ARE TEN KEY FOODS YOU NEED	
Greens	Kale, escarole, spinach, broccoli and cabbage
Whole grains	Brown rice, barley, oatmeal, quinoa, and millet
Berries	Blackberries, blueberries, cranberries, strawberries
Olive oil	Extra virgin, cold-pressed
Tomatoes	Yellow tomatoes are less acidic than red tomatoes
Nuts	Almonds, walnuts, legumes, pistachios, and sunflower seeds
Grapes	Red, green and purple
Fish	Wild Alaskan salmon, cod, halibut, sardines, tilapia
Tea	White and green teas are loaded with antioxidants
Herbs and spices	Turmeric, ginger, garlic, onions, cinnamon, and curry

ALL-STAR FOODS WORTHY OF A STANDING OVATION

First I want to talk to you about the power of fish. I am not referring to the two fish that Jesus used to feed 5,000 people. Rather, I am

Mood-Stabilizing Foods

Chromium - Blood Sugar Stabilizer	Broccoli, grapes, oranges, grains
Folic Acid and B12 for Depression	Rice, beans, oranges, greens, salmon, eggs, milk
Magnesium - Helps PMS and bipolar disorder	Wheat and oat bran, brown rice, nuts, molasses
Omega 3 Fatty Acids - Builds Healthy Brain Cells	Oily fish, walnuts, flaxseed oil
Zinc - for Postpartum Depression	Oysters, lean meats, beans, nuts, oatmeal

referring to the fish that in just a few bites is rich in Omega 3 and good fats. If we were having a fish beauty contest, these would be in the winner's circle:

- Anchovies
- Herring
- Mackerel
- Oysters
- Sable fish
- Sardines
- Wild Alaskan salmon
- Abalone
- Catfish
- Caviar
- Clams
- Crabs
- Crawfish
- Halibut
- Mahi mahi
- Mussels
- Scallops
- Shrimp
- Spot prawns
- Striped bass
- Sturgeon
- Tilapia

ALL STAR VEGGIES AND FRUITS

Some great veggies to keep on hand are carrots, red and green peppers, squash, purple cabbage, eggplant, asparagus, beets, tomatoes, avocados, celery, cucumber, zucchini, pumpkin, radishes, turnips, garlic, leeks, onions, corn, beans, lentils, peas, tofu made from soy beans, potatoes, and sweet potatoes (which are an incredible source of vitamin A and C, fiber, potassium and beta carotene). Skip the gooey and syrupy toppings. Sweet potatoes have integrity on their own. They are wonderful, sweet, and delicious.

Some favorite fruits are oranges, peaches, cantaloupe, grapefruit, honeydew melons, tangerines, apricots, bananas, red and green grapes, kiwi fruit, cranberries, pears, dates, plums, cherries, mango, pineapples, and raisins.

Some noteworthy leafy and cruciferous, gorgeous veggies are kale, collard greens, spinach, bok choy, swiss chard, mustard greens, beet greens, turnip greens, lettuce arugula, lemon balm, endive escarole, broccoli, cabbage, Brussels sprouts, and cauliflower.

We should fall in love with Wholly Fit whole grains. They help protect against cardiovascular disease, type II diabetes and obesity. They also contain healthy fiber and are an incredible source of protein, vitamins, and minerals and they contain healthy phytochemicals. (These are non-nutritive plant chemicals that have protective or disease preventive properties.) There are more than a thousand known phytochemicals. It is well-known that plants produce these chemicals to protect themselves, but recent research demonstrates that they can protect humans against diseases. Some of the well-known phytochemicals are lycopene in tomatoes, isoflavones in soy and flavanoids in fruits. Phytochemicals are not essential nutrients required by the human body for sustaining life, but they will help fight against disease.

Whole grains also contain healthy anti-oxidants. They help you feel full faster so you will eat less. Whole grain fiber is associated with a low risk of colorectal cancer.

On the packaging ingredients, look for 100% whole grain. At least half the grains you consume should come from whole grains. Here are examples of whole grain foods and flours recommended by the whole grain counsel:

- amaranth
- buckwheat
- barley
- corn (this includes whole corn meal and popcorn)
- millet
- oats (this means oatmeal too)
- quinoa
- rice (brown rice and colored rice)
- rye
- sorghum (is also called milo)

After loading your grocery cart with "wonderfoods," go home and make preparations to change your life. Plan your meals ahead of time. Eat more often (five small meals per day). Eat five servings of vegetables and four servings of fruit every day. Switch to whole grains! Be militant and remember the white stuff may cause cancer! Eat two to three servings of calcium-rich foods every day. Eat beans three to five times every week and always, always, always watch your portion sizes.

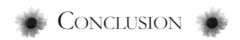# Conclusion

"In order to change we must be sick
and tired of being sick and tired."
Author Unknown

It is beyond comprehension to imagine what would happen if we, as God's people, found wholeness and healing and finally united our hearts together as one body. We would see God's kingdom come and His will be done in us. So, remember to enjoy the path, slow down, take the time to live, reflect, rejoice and renew. Be happy. Don't worry. Simplify your world. Celebrate every chance you get! Do not be afraid to pour your life out and be benevolent and generous to those along the way who may be less fortunate than you. Give something back! In doing so, you will be one of the happiest and healthiest people in the world.

Change is never easy and goes against the grain of human nature; however, it is a vital and necessary process we must all walk through so that we may then explore and conquer new horizons. These new horizons will look different for each of us individually and the challenge will require every ounce of determination we possess, but WE CAN DO IT!!! One of the most important things to remember is to make a plan and then stick with it. Start off by taking small steps and incorporating them into your lifestyle as you can. Remove bad habits and replace them with good habits. Instead of stocking your kitchen with your favorite junk food, fill it with delicious, amazing fruits that will leave you satisfied and energized. Instead of sitting on the couch and doing nothing, get up and walk your poodle, Fifi, around the block. She will love it and so will your body! You could also insert the exercise CD from the back of this book into your disc player (Hint, Hint!!!!) and have a par-tay!!!!!!!!! No one has to see you! Plus, it is such great fun to cut loose and make a ruckus every once in a while.

We must not allow anger, frustration, depression, bitterness and complacency to overcome our minds and steal our joy. Instead, we must process those feelings as they come to us, and once we have trudged through their dense ugliness, we must set our eyes on the promising beauty that lies ahead and walk through a new door. We must fill our minds with positive, happy thoughts, forgive those who would try to steal our peace, and press on toward the joyful life that a healthy mind and body can bring. Together, let's help each other become Wholly Fit!

Fun and Healthy Recipes

Quinoa Stew

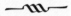

*Quinoa is a whole grain with a texture similar to brown rice, but it is softer, smaller and has a gentle, slightly nutty taste. Quinoa picks up the flavor(s) of whatever you serve it with and is delicious when prepared correctly. This requires a prudent washing and gentle toasting of the grains in order to remove any bitterness from the grain and bring out its nutlike qualities before adding to the boiling water.

Quinoa
1 cup quinoa
Water as needed

In a small stock pot, bring 2 cups of water to a boil. Meanwhile, fill a medium mixing bowl with water, thoroughly submerge 1 cup of quinoa, and then strain with a fine-mesh strainer. Repeat 3 times using fresh, clean water each time.

In a large skillet, gently toast the washed, strained quinoa over a low flame, stirring occasionally until the nutty smell of the grain is detected and it has darkened slightly. This may take up to 10 minutes. If the grains are popping, the heat is too high.

Once quinoa is lightly toasted, add it to the boiling water and reduce to a simmer. Cook 10-15 minutes until all water is absorbed and the round grains sprout tiny little "tails." Strain off any extra cooking liquid and set aside.

Stew
2 large, sweet onions, halved, cut into large dices
2 tbsp. extra-virgin olive oil
1 clove garlic, minced
1/2 lb button mushrooms, cleaned, stems removed, quartered

Quinoa Stew, Con't.

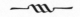

3 large tomatoes, halved, cut into large dices
1 tsp. celery seed
1/2 tsp. ground basil
1/2 tsp. ground oregano
1/2 cup water
1 lb. carrots, cut into large dices
Prepared quinoa
Water as needed
1/4 lb. fresh spinach

In a small stock pot, sauté onions in oil over medium heat until translucent (5-10 minutes). Add garlic and mushrooms. Sauté until liquid is released. Add tomatoes, celery seeds, basil, oregano and water. Bring to a boil, covered. Add carrots, but do not stir.

Cover and simmer over low-medium heat for 30 minutes or until tender.

Grilled Vegetables

1/2 cup lemon juice
1 tbsp. oregano
1 tbsp. crushed garlic
2 lbs assorted fresh vegetables
(I prefer eggplant, zucchini, mushrooms, and onions)

Combine lemon juice, oregano, and garlic. Cut vegetables into large chunks, and onions into wedges. Toss vegetables in lemon and herb mixture. Place them in a single layer on grill or use skewer. Cover and grill 10 to 20 minutes or until tender.

Wholly Fit Artichoke Soup

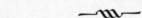

1 tbsp. chicken broth
1 tbsp. olive oil
1 small minced onion
4 minced garlic cloves
1 14 oz. can artichokes,
rinsed, drained and chopped.
2 cups broth or stock
1/2 tsp. dried parsley
1/2 tsp. dried basil
1/2 tsp. dried oregano
Salt to taste.

Cayenne to taste
Fresh lemon juice to taste

Heat the broth and oil in stock
pot over medium heat. Next,
sautee the onion and garlic
until translucent. Then, stir
in the artichokes, broth and
herbs. Add the salt, cayenne
and lemon juice. Cover and
simmer 30 minutes.

Olive Energy Salad

I eat this when I need extra
energy!

1 cup pitted olives, any style
2 lbs. vine-ripened tomatoes,
cubed
1 small onion, diced
1 clove garlic, minced
1 tbsp. fresh lemon juice
1 tbsp. agave nectar or raw
honey
1 head of basil, coarsely
chopped

Salt and pepper to taste
1 tbsp. toasted sesame seeds

In a large mixing bowl, toss
together olives, tomatoes,
onion, garlic, lemon juice,
sweetener, basil, salt, and
pepper. Chill in the refrigerator
for 30 minutes. Spoon into
bowls. Then garnish with
toasted sesame seeds.

Steamed Artichoke
with Spicy Extra-Virgin Olive Oil

2 globe artichokes
1 lemon
1 clove garlic, thinly sliced
Splash of white wine
Pinch of finely ground black
pepper
1/4 cup extra virgin olive oil
1/4 tsp. salt
1/4 tsp. red pepper flakes

Cut off the bottom stems of the artichokes and rub the artichoke bottoms with the lemon. Cut about 2 inches off the top of the artichoke and drizzle lemon juice over the top.

Snip off the pointy ends of each outer leaf with scissors. This will keep you from getting stung later when the artichoke is ready to eat.

Using a stock pot big enough to fit and cover two artichokes, bring 3 inches of water to a boil. Add the garlic, wine, and pepper. Using tongs, carefully place artichokes top down

into the pot. Simmer over fork to check for doneness. If it is tender, the artichoke is cooked. Another indicator of a fully cooked artichoke is leaves that pull off easily. Using tongs, remove artichokes from the pot and set upright on a serving plate.

In a dipping bowl, whisk together olive oil, salt and red pepper flakes.

To eat the artichoke, pull the leaves and dip the bottom tender part into the dipping oil and, using your teeth, pull off the tender "meat" from the bottom part of the leaves. Do not eat the rough tops. As more leaves come off, those toward the inside are more tender and the whole leaf can be eaten. Toward the heart of the artichoke, you will see fuzz. This should be scraped off with a spoon. What remains is the best part of all - the center or "heart" of the artichoke.

Grilled Lemon-Garlic Chicken
—w—

1 tsp. grated lemon zest
1/3 cup freshly squeezed
lemon juice
1/4 cut extra-virgin olive oil
2 tbsp. Dijon mustard
Freshly ground pepper to taste
2 garlic cloves, pressed
4 skinless, boneless chicken
breast halves.
10-12 ounces spinach,
stemmed and coarsely
chopped.
Nasturtium blossoms and/or
slivered yellow bell peppers
for garnish.

In a small bowl, whisk together
the lemon zest, juice, oil,
mustard, and pepper. Pour
about 2/3 of the mixture into a
bowl large enough to hold the
chicken. Reserve the remaining
dressing. Add the garlic to the
bowl, then add the chicken
and toss to coat. Cover and
marinate for one hour at room
temperature, or refrigerate for
2 to 24 hours.

Light a fire in a charcoal or gas
grill. If the chicken has been
refrigerated, remove it from the
refrigerator 30 minutes before
cooking. Cook the chicken
over a medium-hot fire for 3
to 4 minutes per side, or until
opaque throughout.

In a covered steamer or
saucepan, steam the spinach
over boiling water just until
wilted, about 1 minute. Toss
with the reserved dressing.
Divide the spinach among 4
dinner plates and top with a
chicken breast half. Garnish
with nasturtiums and/or yellow
bell pepper slivers.

Grilled Shrimp
with Mustard Green Salsa

1 lb. large shrimp, peeled and de-veined, tails left on
4 tbsp. extra-virgin olive oil
Freshly ground pepper to taste
1 tbsp. mustard seeds
1 lb. mustard greens, stemmed and coarsely chopped
4 garlic cloves, chopped
1/2 cup fresh lemon juice
1 tbsp. grated lemon zest
2 tbsp. Dijon mustard
1/4 cup low-fat mayonnaise
Salt to taste
Lemon zest curls for garnish

Light a fire in a gas or charcoal grill. In a medium bowl, toss the shrimp with 1 tbsp. of the oil and pepper. Set aside.

In a sauté pan, sauté the mustard seeds over medium-high heat until fragrant, stirring constantly. Transfer the greens to a blender or food processor. Add the lemon juice and zest, mustard, mayonnaise, salt and pepper to taste. Blend until smooth. Place the shrimp in a small bowl, add the remaining 2 tbsp. oil, and toss until lightly coated. Skewer the shrimp and grill over white-hot coals until pink and opaque, 1 to 2 minutes per side.

Spoon the salsa in the center of each serving plate and surround with shrimp. Top each shrimp with a lemon zest curl.

Beans and Bitter Greens

2 tbsp. extra-virgin olive oil
1 bunch dandelion, mustard,
or turnip greens (10 to 12
ounces), stemmed and cut
into 1/2-inch ribbons
4 garlic cloves, thinly sliced
2 tbsp. mirin (sweet sake) or
dry sherry
2 tbsp. fresh lemon juice
1 tbsp. Dijon mustard
1/2 cup cooked garbanzo
beans, drained and rinsed
1/4 cup finely slivered red bell
pepper or diced tomato
Salt and freshly ground pepper
to taste

In a large skillet or sauté
pan, heat 1 tbsp. of oil over
medium-high heat. Add the
greens and garlic and sauté
for 1 minute. Lower heat. Add
the mirin (or dry sherry), cover
and simmer for 10 minutes.
Remove from heat.

In a small bowl, whisk together
the lemon juice, mustard, and
remaining 1 tbsp of oil. Add
to the greens along with the
remaining ingredients. Toss
thoroughly.

Oven Potato Chips

Pre heat oven to 450 degrees. Use a non stick cookie sheet or
a cookie sheet sprayed with organic olive oil non stick spray.
Scrub potatoes and slice them. Place potato slices (one layer
only) on cookie sheet. Sprinkle with garlic powder and garlic
pepper. Bake 5 min; turn potatoes and cook till crisp.

Spicy Pecan Halibut
with Asparagus

—⚊⚊—

Spiced Nuts
1 tbsp. olive oil
1/2 cup chopped pecan pieces
1/2 tsp. cayenne pepper
1/2 tsp. ground cumin
1/2 tsp. salt

Balsamic Glaze
1 cup balsamic vinegar
2 tbsp. packed, brown sugar
1/4 tsp. cayenne pepper

3 tbsp. pure olive oil
Four 8-oz halibut steaks, each 1 1/2 inches thick
Salt and freshly ground pepper to taste
2 tsp. canola oil
1 lb. baby asparagus spears, trimmed

To make the spiced nuts: In a small sauté pan or skillet, heat the oil over low heat. Add the pecans, cayenne, cumin, and salt and sauté until the nuts are lightly toasted. Set aside.

To make the glaze: Combine the vinegar, brown sugar, and cayenne in a small saucepan. Bring to a boil, reduce to a simmer, and cook to reduce to a thick glaze. Set aside.

Preheat the oven to 350 °F. In a large skillet, heat the olive oil over high heat until almost smoking. Season the fish with salt and pepper and sear for 2 to 3 minutes on each side. Transfer the fish to a warm platter and set aside. In the same skillet, heat the canola oil over medium-high heat and sauté the asparagus, stirring constantly for 3 to 4 minutes or until crisp-tender.

Drizzle the balsamic glaze over the fish, sprinkle with the spiced nuts, and garnish with a fan of asparagus.

Chicken and Asparagus Stir Fry

4 boneless, skinless chicken breasts
2 tbsp. of crushed garlic
1/2 medium, yellow onion chopped
1 lb. of mushrooms thinly sliced
1 can water chestnuts
1 lbs of asparagus cut off tough ends and cut into two inch pieces
1 cup of non fat, low sodium chicken broth
1 half cup white wine

Heat a nonstick wok, add chicken and garlic and stir fry until chicken is almost done Remove the chicken. Add mushrooms, onions, chicken broth, white wine, and asparagus.

Stir fry for 3 minutes. Add water chestnuts and then add chicken. Season with salt and pepper as desired

Poached Chicken

4 boneless skinless chicken breasts
1 cup rice vinegar
1 tbsp. crushed fresh ginger root
1 cup non fat, low sodium chicken broth
2 tbsp. crushed garlic
2 sprigs of basil, chopped

Place ingredients in shallow pan, except basil. Bring the liquid to a boil. Cover and simmer over low heat for 25 minutes. Add chopped basil. Simmer 5 more minutes. Then serve over brown rice.

Fruity Yogurt
—∿—

1 cup plain organic yogurt (I like Nancy's organic yogurt)
1 cup mixed berries
1 cup papaya or mango
1 tbsp. milled or ground flax seed
a dash of ground cinnamon

Combine all ingredients, except cinnamon. Spoon into parfait glasses and sprinkle with cinnamon. Chill before serving.

Fruit Shake
—∿—

1 lemon
1 tbsp. Stevia or Lakanto (sugar substitute)
4 cups ice
1 cup berries
1/2 cup water

Squeeze juice from lemon and pour into blender. Add sweetener, fruit and two cups of ice. Blend to desired consistency. Add in last two cups of ice and water.

Broiled Cinnamon Grapefruit
—∿—

1 grapefruit (ruby red is the best)
Dash of cinnamon
1 tsp of Stevia or Lakanto (sugar substitute)

Peel the grapefruit. Mix grapefruit pieces with cinnamon and sugar substitute.

Eat cold or if desired, or broil until the sugar substitute caramelizes.

Avocado and Bean Burrito
—m—

2 cups shredded romaine
lettuce
2 tbsp. yellow onions,
chopped
1/2 medium avocado, peeled,
pitted and chopped
2 tbsp. chopped cilantro
4 tbsp. chunky salsa
1/2 cup nonfat vegetarian
refried beans
2 sprouted corn tortillas

Mix lettuce, onion, avocado,
cilantro and salsa until
vegetables are evenly coated.
Smear half of the beans on
each tortilla. Fill with vegetable
mixture and wrap burrito style.

Dilled Egg Salad on Spinach
—m—

4 eggs
2 tbsp. finely chopped
scallions
2 tbsp. finely chopped fresh
dill
2 tbsp. soy mayonnaise
1 pinch of sea salt
1 dash freshly ground black
pepper
3 cups baby spinach
1 large, red apple cut into
wedges

Place eggs in medium
saucepan and cover with
cold water. Bring to a boil
then remove from heat and let
stand 15 minutes. Drain eggs
and place in cold water to
chill. Then peel off eggshells.
Combine eggs, scallions,
dill, mayo, mustard, salt and
pepper in medium bowl and
toss gently. Arrange greens
and apples on salad plate. Top
with prepared egg salad.

Cashew Shrimp Lettuce Wraps

1/2 cup natural cashew butter
1 tbsp. coconut milk
3 tbsp. lime juice
1/4 tsp. chili powder
1/2 lb. cooked shrimp, thawed if frozen
1/4 cup chopped scallions
1/2 cup shredded carrots
1/2 cup bean sprouts, washed and drained
1/2 cup cucumber, seeded and diced
1/4 cup sesame seeds
1 tbsp. grated, fresh ginger
1/2 tbsp. low sodium soy sauce
2 tbsp. lime juice
1/4 cup rice vinegar

6 large leaves Boston lettuce, washed

In small bowl, whip cashew butter, 3 tbsp. lime juice and chili powder. In large bowl, combine shrimp, scallions, carrots, bean sprouts, cucumber, sesame seeds, ginger, soy, 2 tbsp. lime juice and vinegar. Mix well and let flavors marinate in refrigerator for 20 minutes. Divide cashew sauce and shrimp/vegetable mixture in center of each leaf and wrap lettuce around filling. Wrap and serve.

Sweet Green Smoothie

2 bananas, peeled
3 oranges, peeled and quartered
1 head of romaine lettuce
4 cups cold water

Add ingredients to blender in this order: bananas, oranges, then romaine. Add water and blend on medium-high until smooth. Serve immediately.

Banana Split for Kiddos!

—∿—

1 banana
2 tbsp. fruit preserves
2 tbsp. Cool Whip
Lettuce and raisins

Split banana down the center and place on a bed of lettuce. Spread on fruit preserves and Cool Whip. Top with raisins.

Fruit Salad for Kiddos!

—∿—

4 cups of your child's favorite fruit - melons, apples, oranges, bananas, etc.
1-2 cups vanilla yogurt

Mix fruit together in a bowl. Add yogurt. Cool in refrigerator for at least one hour before serving.

Tropical Fruit Smoothie

—∿—

1 mango, peeled and seeded
1 papaya, peeled and seeded
1 banana, peeled
1 orange, peeled
5 ice cubes

Blend all ingredients in a blender until smooth. Serve immediately.

Chinese Cabbage Salad

1/2 cup smooth, natural
peanut butter
1/2 cup hot water
1/2 cup plus 1 tbsp. rice
vinegar
3 tbsp. packed brown sugar
1/2 tsp. salt
1 tbsp. low sodium soy sauce
1 tsp. Asian sesame oil
7 to 8 cups green cabbage,
including outer leaves,
shredded
Cayenne pepper to taste
4 oz. unsalted, roasted
peanuts, crushed
3 whole, green onions,
chopped

In large bowl, mix peanut
butter and hot water into
smooth paste. Add vinegar,
sugar, salt, soy sauce and
sesame oil. Mix thoroughly.
Add cabbage one cup at a
time, mixing thoroughly with
each added cup. Sprinkle
with cayenne to taste and mix
again. Cover and refrigerate 4
to 24 hours. Stir several times
while chilling. Sprinkle w/
chopped peanuts and green
onions just before serving.

Creamed Spinach

Instead of relying on butter and cream, create the silky texture of this childhood favorite with lowfat milk and reduced fat cream cheese, one tbsp. olive oil, one finely chopped onion, one chopped garlic clove, kosher salt and black pepper, ½ 8 oz. bar reduced fat cream cheese

¾ cup 1% milk
2 10 oz pkg's frozen spinach, thawed
Pinch of nutmeg

Heat oil in large skillet over medium heat. Add onion, garlic, salt, pepper. Cook 6 to 7 minutes, stirring until soft. Add cream cheese and milk and cook. Stir until cream cheese is melted. Squeeze any excess liquid out of spinach. Add spinach to sauce. Cook 3 to 4 minutes until heated through and thickened. Sprinkle with nutmeg.

Iceberg Wedge
with Blue Cheese Dressing

½ cup buttermilk
2 tbsp reduced fat sour cream
4 tbsp crumbled blue cheese
1 head iceberg lettuce, quartered
Black garlic pepper

In small bowl, whip together, buttermilk, sour cream and 3 tbsp blue cheese. Divide lettuce among plates and spoon dressing over the top Sprinkle with remaining tbsp of blue cheese and pepper.

Green Beans
with Mushrooms and Crispy Onion Rings

½ small red onion, cut into thin rings and separated
2 tbsp. flour
½ Kosher salt and ½ tsp black pepper
3 tbsp olive oil
8 oz button mushrooms
1 cup 1 % milk
1 lb frozen green beans, thawed

In a bowl, toss onion w/ one tbsp of flour and dash of salt. Heat ½ of oil in large skillet over medium heat. Cook onion until golden brown. Wipe out skillet and heat remaining oil over medium high heat. Cook mushrooms 5 to 6 minutes until tender. Reduce heat to medium. Sprinkle remaining flour over mushrooms and cook, stirring for one minute. Add milk, remaining salt and pepper. Simmer, stirring 1 to 2 minutes until mixture thickens. Add beans, cook until heated through. Top with onions.

All-Time Favorite Meatloaf

1/3 cup egg substitute
1 can 6 0z. tomato paste, divided
2 tbsp Dijon mustard
2 tsp prepared horseradish (divided)
½ cup quick cooking oats
1 envelope onion soup mix
1 ½ tsp garlic powder
1 tsp steak seasoning
1 lb. lean ground beef
½ lb lean ground turkey
1 tsp water

In large bowl, combine egg substitute, ½ cup tomato paste, mustard, 1 tsp horseradish, oats, soup mix, garlic powder and steak seasoning. Crumble beef and turkey over mixture and mix well. Shape into loaf and put into 11 x 7 baking dish coated w/ cooking spray. Combine water, tomato paste and horseradish. Add 2 tsp water. Spread over meatloaf. Bake uncovered at 350 for 45 to 55 minutes.

Wholly Wonderful Strawberry Rhubarb Crunch

—ɱ—

½ cup sugar or Stevia or Lekanto
2 tbsp corn starch
2 ½ cup cliced, fresh straw
2 cups diced rhubarb (frozen or fresh)
1 tsp vanilla extract
2/3 cup all purpose flour
½ cup quick cooking oats
1/4 cup brown sugar
½ tsp ground cinnamon
¼ cup cooled butter

In large saucepan, combine sugar and cornstarch. Stir in straws and rubarb till blended. Bring to boil. Cook and stir 1 to 2 minutes or until thickens. Remove from heat. Stir in vanilla. Pour into 8 inch baking dish coated with cooking spray. In small bowl, combine flour, oats, brown sugar and cinnamon. Cut in butter until crumbly. Sprinkle over fruit mixture. Bake at 350 for 25 to 30 minutes or until filling is bubbly and topping is golden brown. Serve w/ shipped topping or cream if desired (unless ou are trying to restrict calories – then skip the whipped cream.

Old-Fashioned Strawberry Pie

—⟋⟍—

1 pkg 3 oz cook and serve vanilla pudding mix
1 ½ cups of water
1 tsp lemon juice
1 pkg 3 oz sugar free strawberry gelatin
½ cup boiling water
4 cups sliced fresh strawberries
3 oz reduced fat cream cheese
2 cups reduced fat whipped topping, divided
1 tsp. vanilla extract
8 fresh, whole strawberries

First, bake pie crust and set aside. Next, in a small saucepan combine pudding mix, water and lemon juice. Cook and stir over medium heat until it comes to a boil. Then cook, stirring an additional 1 to 2 minutes longer until it thickens. Remove from heat and set aside.

Dissolve gelatin in water, stir in pudding mixture and fold in sliced strawberries. Transfer to pastry crust, cover and refrigerate 30 minutes.

Topping

In a small bowl, beat cream cheese, ½ cup whipped topping and vanilla until smooth. Fold in the rest of whipped topping. Pipe the topping around the edge of pie and garnish with whole strawberries. Refrigerate at least one hour before serving.

7-day fabulous, healthy way to lose weight quickly for your birthday!!!!

This diet is fast. The secret lies within the principle that you will burn more calories than you take in while it flushes your system of impurities.

- 3 large bunches green onions
- 1 large can of beef or chicken broth (no fat)
- 1 pkg. Lipton Soup mix (chicken noodle) - use entire package
- 1 bunch of celery
- 2 cans (or fresh) green beans
- 2 lbs. carrots
- 2 green bell peppers

Cut veggies in small to medium pieces and cover with water. Boil fast for 10 minutes, reduce heat and add broth and package of Lipton soup mix. Season with salt and pepper, curry, chili powder, hot sauce or Worcestershire sauce. Reduce to simmer and continue to cook until veggies are just tender. Chop fresh parsley or cilantro and add after you turn off heat if desired.

This soup can be eaten anytime you are hungry during the week. Eat as much as you want, whenever you want. This soup will not add calories. The more you eat, the more you will lose. You may want to fill a thermos in the morning if you will be away during the day.

Drinks

- Unsweetened juices
- Tea (including herbal)
- Coffee
- Cranberry juice
- Skim milk
- Water, water, water

Day One

Any fruit (except bananas). Cantaloupes and watermelon are lower in calories than most other fruits. Eat only soup and fruit today.

Day Two

All vegetables. Eat until you are stuffed with fresh, raw, cooked or canned veggies. Try to eat green, leafy veggies and stay away from dry beans, peas or corn. Eat veggies along with the soup. At dinnertime, reward yourself with a big baked potato and butter. Do not eat any fruits today.

Day Three

Eat all the soup, fruit and veggies you want. Do not eat a baked potato. If you have eaten as above for three days and not cheated, you should find that you have lost 5-7 pounds.

Day Four

Bananas and skim milk: eat at least 3 bananas and drink as much skim milk as you can today, along with the soup. Bananas are high in calories and carbohydrates, as is the milk but on this particular day, your body will need the potassium and carbs. Proteins and calcium to lessen the cravings for sweets.

Day Five

Beef and tomatoes: you may have 10 to 20 ounces of beef and a can of tomatoes, or as many as 6 tomatoes on this day. Eat the soup at least once today.

Day Six

Beef and veggies: eat to your heart's content of the beef and veggies today. You can even have 2-3 steaks if you like, with leafy, green veggies but no baked potato. Be sure to eat the soup at least once today.

Day Seven

Brown rice, unsweetened fruit juice and veggies. Again, be sure to stuff yourself and eat the soup. You can add cooked veggies to your rice if you wish. By the end of the 7th day, if you have not cheated on this diet, you should have lost 10 to 17 pounds. If you have lost more than 17 pounds, stay off the diet for two days before resuming the diet again.

Due to the variety of digestive systems in individuals, this diet will affect everyone differently. After day three, you will have more energy than when you began if you do not cheat. After being on the diet for several days, you will find that your bowel movements have changed. Eat a cup of bran or fiber. Although you can have black coffee with this diet, you may find that you do not need caffeine after the third day.

The basic fat burning soup can be eaten anytime you feel hungry during the seven days . Eat as much as you wish. Remember the more you eat, the more you will lose. You can eat broiled, boiled or baked chicken instead of the beef. Absolutely no skin on the chicken. If you prefer, you can substitute broiled fish for the beef on only one of the beef days. You need the high protein in the beef for the other days.

No bread, alcohol, carbonated drinks (including diet drinks). Remember, absolutely no fried foods. Drink plenty of water (at least 6 to 8 glasses per day) as well as any combination of black coffee, unsweetened fruit drinks, cranberry juice and skim milk.

We are not sure why this diet is "Secret" but that it may have been used for overweight heart patients in order to lose weight rapidly for health reasons. Obviously, use your best judgment in undertaking any diet regime. PLEASE CONSULT YOUR PHYSICIAN FIRST.

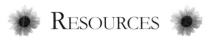

RESOURCES

www.revolutionhealth.com/healthy-living/food-nutrition/food-basics/essential-nutrients/bottled-water

Mayo Clinic Healthy Weight for Everybody, Donald Hensrud and The Mayo Clinic

Adult BMI and Calorie Calculator. www.bcm.edu/cnrs/caloriesneed.htm

Body Mass index (BMI) Calculator, U.S. Centers for Disease Control and Prevention. www.cdc.gov/nccdphp/dnpa/bmi/calc-bmi.htm.

U.S. Government Food and Nutrition Information: www.nutrition.gov

U.S. Dietary Guidelines for Americans. www.health.gov

Whole Grain Council. www.wholegrainscouncil.org

World Health Organization Report "Diet, Nutrition and the Prevention of Chronic Diseases." www.fao.org/docrep/005/ac911E/ac911e00.htm

Shoppers Guide to Pesticides in Produce. www.foodnews.org/pdf/ewg_pesticide.pdf;

www.foodnews.org/index.php

Children's Ads Show Lots of Junk. Kevin Freking Associated Press Newswires, March 28, 2007.

Eat Food, Not Too Much. Michael Pollan, "Unhappy Meals" *New York Times Magazine*, January 28, 2007.

Tara Parker-Pope "Fat Helps You Absorb Vegetables and Nutrients" *The Wall Street Journal*, August 13, 2006

Calories Burned by Walking. R.J. Ignelzi "Fitness Walking" *The San Diego Union Tribune*, October 31, 2006.

We Ought to Think of Soft Drinks as a Treat. Bonnie Liebman, Morning Star Nutrition Action Health Letter, January 1, 2007.

The Fast Track One-Day Detox Diet, Ann Louise Gittleman, Ph.D., C.N.S.

Young Skin for Life, Julie Davis and Editors of *Prevention Magazine*

137

The Body Ecology Diet, Donna Gates. www.bodyecologydiet.com

Nutrition Almanac, 6th Edition, John D. Kirschmann and Nutrition Search, Inc.

"Our Super-Sized Kids," *Time Magazine*, Special Health Issue, June 23, 2008

The Owner's Manual, Michael F. Roizen, M.D. and Mehmet C. Oz, M.D.

Nutrition Almanac, 6th Edition. "Hair Problems"

The Well Being Journal, May - June 2008

More Natural Cures Revealed, Kevin Trudeau

The Food Bible, Gillian McKeith

King James Version

New International Version

The Amplified Version

The Message

Notes

Notes

Notes

Notes

Notes

For information on these products and to order,
please visit www.nancygrandquist.com.

BOOKS
True Tales of Jean Norene
a children's book by Heidi King
Priceless Garments by Nancy Grandquist

Soon to be released...
Voice of Wisdom
(a collection of true life stories
about women and their indelible influences)

CDs
Mystery by Heidi King
My Promise Land by Nancy Grandquist
Come Lord Jesus by Nancy Grandquist
Songs for Those We Love by Nancy Grandquist
Somebody Special by Nancy Grandquist
Whispering Wonders by Nancy Grandquist
Our God is One by Nancy Grandquist
Truth Shall Triumph by Nancy Grandquist
Get Yourself Ready by Nancy Grandquist
Heart Worship by Nancy Grandquist
A Christmas Blessing by Nancy Grandquist
704 Tupper Street by Nancy Grandquist
Testify by Nancy Grandquist